IODINE HEALING

HANDBOOK

A Step-by-Step Guide to Restoring Thyroid Health, Detoxing Your Body, Boosting Immunity, and Thriving with More Energy

Arden Harper

TABLE OF CONTENT

Introduction 8

    Why Iodine Matters in Today's World 8

PART 1: THE BASICS OF IODINE 10

Chapter 1: Understanding Iodine's Health Role.............................. 10

    Iodine: The Forgotten Nutrient 10

    How Iodine Works in Your Body 12

    Are You Deficient in Iodine? 13

Chapter 2: Common Myths About Iodine 16

    The Truth About Iodized Salt.. 16

    Debunking Iodophobia... 17

    Is Iodine Dangerous in Large Doses? 19

Part 2: Practical Guide to Using Iodine 21

Chapter 3: Choosing and Using the Right Iodine........................... 22

    Types of Iodine Supplements 22

    Which Iodine Is Right for You?.. 24

    Iodine in Food Sources.. 26

Chapter 4: Safely Incorporating Iodine 28

    Step-by-Step Dosage Guidelines 28

    Adapting Iodine for Thyroid, Detox, and Energy 30

    Avoiding Overuse and Side Effects 31

Chapter 5: Supporting Iodine with Nutrients 34

    The Iodine-Selenium Connection 34

    Other Key Nutrients: Magnesium, Zinc, Vitamin D 36

    Salt Loading for Bromide Detox.. 37

PART 3: Healing with Iodine 39

Chapter 6: Iodine and Thyroid Health 40

    Healing Hypothyroidism..40

    Autoimmune Thyroid Disorders 42

    Iodine's Role in Thyroid Cancer Prevention 44

Chapter 7: Detoxing Your Body with Iodine...................................... 46

    Detoxing Heavy Metals with Iodine... 46

    Fluoride and Bromide Detox... 48

    Creating a Detox Plan 49

Chapter 8: Boosting Immunity and Energy 52

    Strengthening Your Immune System.. 52

    Reclaiming Your Energy.. 54

    Brain Function and Mental Clarity 56

PART 4: Special Applications of Iodine... 58

Chapter 9: Iodine for Women's Health... 58

    Breast Health and Hormonal Balance 58

    Iodine During Pregnancy 60

Chapter 10: Iodine for Men's Health 62

    Prostate Health and Iodine's Role 62

    Testosterone and Vitality 64

Chapter 11: Iodine for Youth Health.. 66

    Brain Development Support 66

    ADHD and Autism: Iodine's Neurobehavioral Benefits................... 68

    Safe Doses for Kids 70

Chapter 12: Preventing and Treating Cancer with Iodine................. 72

Iodine and Breast Cancer Prevention 72

Skin Cancer Applications 74

Part 5: Resources and Tools 76

Chapter 13: FAQs About Iodine 76

Common Concerns 76

Chapter 14: Advanced Protocols and Testing 79

Why Personalization Matters 79

Types of Detox Programs 80

Light Detox for Beginners 80

Moderate Detox with Lugol's and Nutritional Support 82

Intensive Detox for Deep Toxin Removal 83

Managing Detox Symptoms 85

Common Symptoms 85

Relief Strategies 87

When to Stop... 88

Practical Detox Tools 90

Checklist for Choosing the Right Protocol 90

Tracking Your Progress 92

Chapter 15: Iodine-Rich Diet Recipes... 94

Simple Iodine-Rich Recipes 94

Meal Plans for Thyroid and Detox 97

Thyroid-Boosting Breakfast Plan 97

Detoxifying Lunch Plan 99

Iodine-Rich Dinner Plan... 101

Energy-Enhancing Snack Plan 103

Immune-Boosting Meal Plan.. 105

Metabolism-Revving Breakfast Plan..107

Cleansing Lunch Plan 109

Nutrient-Dense Dinner Plan 111

Hydration-Focused Snack Plan 113

Balanced Meal Plan for Thyroid Health... 115

Conclusion... 117

Thriving with Iodine.. 117

Appendices and References 119

Appendix A: Food Sources of Iodine Chart 119

Appendix B: Iodine Supplement Comparison Table 120

Glossary: Iodine Terms and Concepts Explained.. 121

Introduction

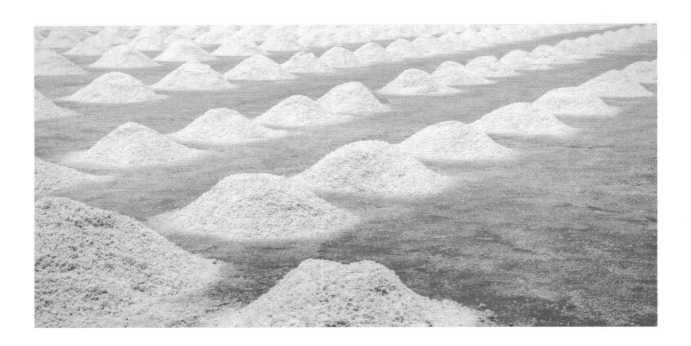

Why Iodine Matters in Today's World

In the landscape of modern health, the significance of iodine cannot be overstated. This essential mineral plays a pivotal role in the functioning of the thyroid gland, which in turn regulates metabolism, energy levels, and overall bodily functions. Despite its critical importance, iodine deficiency has become a widespread issue, affecting millions of individuals worldwide. The reasons behind this deficiency are multifaceted, including dietary changes, soil depletion, and the prevalence of processed foods low in essential nutrients.

Iodine's role extends beyond thyroid health; it is instrumental in detoxifying the body from harmful substances such as heavy metals and environmental toxins. Additionally, it boosts the immune system, making it a key player in fighting infections and maintaining overall health. The body's requirement for iodine increases in certain life stages, such as pregnancy and adolescence, highlighting the need for a conscious effort to ensure adequate intake.

The modern diet, often lacking in fresh, nutrient-rich foods, typically does not provide sufficient amounts of iodine. Seafood and seaweed are among the richest natural sources, yet their consumption is limited in many diets. Furthermore, the reliance on table salt for iodine intake is misguided; the processing of salt reduces its iodine content, and high sodium intake can lead to other health issues.

Recognizing the signs of iodine deficiency is crucial for addressing this hidden epidemic. Symptoms can range from fatigue and weight gain to more severe health conditions such as goiter and cognitive impairments. Simple tests and assessments can help determine iodine levels, offering a pathway to correction through diet and supplementation.

The path to restoring iodine levels and reaping its health benefits involves a multifaceted approach. Incorporating iodine-rich foods into the diet, understanding the different forms of iodine supplements, and tailoring intake to individual needs are essential steps. It is also important to consider the synergy between iodine and other nutrients, such as selenium, for optimal thyroid function and health.

As we delve deeper into the practical applications of iodine in subsequent chapters, remember that the goal is not just to address deficiency but to harness the full spectrum of benefits iodine offers. From detoxification and immunity boosting to enhancing energy levels and preventing chronic diseases, iodine is a cornerstone of a holistic approach to health. The journey to understanding and utilizing this vital nutrient is a testament to the power of informed, proactive health choices in today's world.

PART 1: THE BASICS OF IODINE

Chapter 1: Understanding Iodine's Health Role

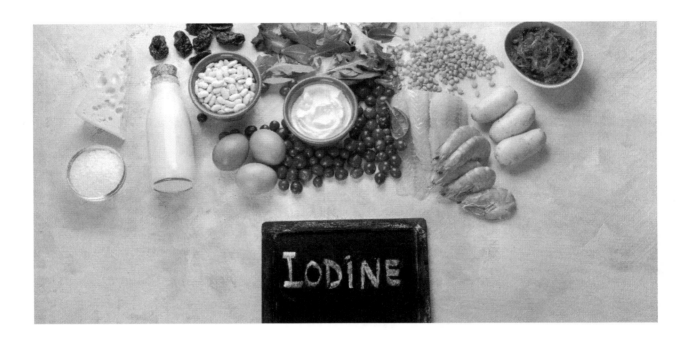

Iodine: The Forgotten Nutrient

The decline in dietary iodine over recent decades is alarming, given its critical role in health. Historically, populations living near oceans consumed ample amounts of iodine through seafood and seaweeds. However, with the shift towards industrial agriculture and processed foods, the natural sources of this vital nutrient have been significantly reduced in the average diet. The soil in many areas, once rich in minerals, has been depleted of iodine due to over-farming and environmental pollutants, further diminishing the iodine content of fruits and vegetables.

In the early 20th century, recognizing the widespread issue of goiter (an enlarged thyroid gland due to iodine deficiency), the United States and several other countries began iodizing table salt. This public health measure significantly reduced the prevalence of goiter and other iodine deficiency disorders. Yet, the reliance on iodized salt has led to a misconception that it alone can provide sufficient iodine. Many people, in an effort to reduce sodium intake for cardiovascular health, have decreased their consumption of table salt, inadvertently lowering their iodine intake as well. Moreover, the form of iodine used in table salt is not always fully bioavailable, and the processing of salt can strip away some of its nutritional value.

The modern diet, characterized by high intakes of processed foods, sugars, and unhealthy fats, often lacks nutrient-dense foods such as fish, seaweed, and vegetables, which are natural sources of iodine. Additionally, certain compounds found in processed foods, such as bromide (used as a dough conditioner) and fluoride (added to drinking water), can interfere with iodine absorption and utilization in the body, exacerbating the problem of deficiency.

To counteract this decline, it is crucial to reintroduce natural sources of iodine into the diet. Seafood, particularly deep-sea fish and seaweeds like kelp, are excellent sources. Dairy products and eggs can also contribute to iodine intake, depending on the iodine content of the feed and soil where the animals are raised. For those with dietary restrictions or who do not consume enough of these foods, iodine supplements, such as Lugol's solution or potassium iodide tablets, can be effective when used under the guidance of a healthcare professional.

Understanding the importance of iodine and recognizing the signs of deficiency are the first steps toward correcting this nutrient shortfall. Symptoms of iodine deficiency can be subtle and often go unnoticed, such as fatigue, weight gain, and feeling cold. More severe consequences include developmental issues in children, decreased fertility, and an increased risk of thyroid disease.

Incorporating a variety of iodine-rich foods into meals and being mindful of factors that can inhibit iodine absorption are practical strategies to ensure adequate intake. For those considering supplementation, it is essential to start with low doses and adjust based on individual needs and response, under the supervision of a healthcare provider. Monitoring iodine levels through urinary iodine concentration tests can provide valuable feedback on one's iodine status and guide dietary and supplementation practices.

As the diet continues to evolve in the modern world, the role of iodine should not be underestimated. By making informed choices about food and supplementation, individuals can support their thyroid health, detoxification processes, immune function, and overall well-being.

How Iodine Works in Your Body

Iodine plays a crucial role in the human body, primarily through its impact on the thyroid gland, cellular energy production, and detoxification processes. The thyroid gland, located at the base of the neck, is responsible for producing hormones that regulate metabolism, growth, and body temperature. For the thyroid to synthesize these hormones, iodine is essential. The body absorbs iodine from dietary sources, converting it into the thyroid hormones thyroxine (T4) and triiodothyronine (T3). These hormones are then released into the bloodstream, where they are transported to cells throughout the body, influencing metabolism, brain development, and bone maintenance.

Cellular energy production is another critical area where iodine exerts its influence. Mitochondria, the energy powerhouses of the cell, require thyroid hormones to regulate cellular metabolism. These hormones adjust the rate at which cells convert nutrients into energy, thus playing a vital role in maintaining energy levels. Adequate levels of iodine ensure that the thyroid gland can produce the hormones necessary for optimal mitochondrial function and energy production.

Detoxification is an often-overlooked aspect of iodine's role in the body. Iodine contributes to the body's detoxification processes by supporting the elimination of toxins, including heavy metals and certain chemicals. It competes with toxic elements like fluoride, bromide, and chlorine, which can inhibit thyroid function, thus preventing their accumulation in the thyroid gland and promoting their excretion. Additionally, iodine has antioxidant properties that help protect cells from oxidative stress, a byproduct of detoxification.

The relationship between iodine and **selenium** is also worth noting. Selenium, an essential trace element, works synergistically with iodine. It is crucial for the conversion of T4 into the more active T3 hormone and for protecting the thyroid gland from oxidative damage during hormone production. This interplay highlights the importance of a balanced intake of both nutrients to support thyroid health and efficient detoxification.

For individuals with iodine deficiency, the body's ability to produce thyroid hormones is compromised, leading to a range of health issues, including hypothyroidism, goiter, and impaired cognitive function. Ensuring adequate iodine intake through diet or supplementation can help maintain thyroid health, support detoxification, and enhance energy metabolism.

It is important for health-conscious adults to recognize the signs of iodine deficiency and understand the sources of iodine, including seafood, dairy products, and iodine-fortified foods. For those who cannot meet their iodine needs through diet alone, iodine supplements may be an option, though it is advisable to consult with a healthcare provider to determine the appropriate dosage and form of iodine supplementation.

In summary, iodine's role in the body extends far beyond thyroid health. It is integral to energy production at the cellular level and plays a vital role in the body's natural detoxification processes. By ensuring adequate iodine intake, individuals can support their overall health and well-being.

Are You Deficient in Iodine?

Recognizing the signs of iodine deficiency is paramount for anyone concerned about their thyroid health and overall well-being. The body's need for this essential mineral is often underestimated, yet its absence can lead to a myriad of health issues that affect daily life significantly. Identifying deficiency early can help mitigate these problems through dietary changes or supplementation. Here are the signs and simple tests to assess iodine levels:

Signs of Iodine Deficiency:

- **Fatigue and Weakness:** A pervasive sense of tiredness that does not improve with rest could indicate low levels of thyroid hormones, often due to insufficient iodine.

- **Unexpected Weight Gain:** Unexplained weight gain can be a sign of a slowed metabolism, a common symptom of iodine deficiency affecting thyroid function.

- **Hair Loss:** The thyroid hormones, supported by iodine, play a key role in hair follicle regeneration. A deficiency may result in noticeable hair thinning or loss.

- **Dry, Flaky Skin:** Since iodine aids in skin regeneration, a deficiency can lead to dry, flaky skin due to slowed cellular turnover.

- **Feeling Colder than Usual:** If you find yourself feeling unusually cold, it could be due to a decrease in thyroid hormone production, affecting your body's temperature regulation.

- **Swelling in the Neck:** A visible swelling or enlargement in the neck, known as a goiter, can indicate an iodine deficiency. The thyroid gland swells in an attempt to absorb more iodine from the bloodstream.

Simple Tests to Assess Iodine Levels:

1. **Urine Test:** The most straightforward method to evaluate iodine levels is through a urinary iodine concentration test. This test measures the amount of iodine excreted in the urine, reflecting the body's iodine status. It's widely used due to its simplicity and effectiveness.

2. **Iodine Patch Test:** This home test involves applying a small amount of iodine tincture to the skin and observing how quickly it fades. A faster-than-expected fading might suggest a deficiency, although this test is not as reliable as urinary testing and should not be used as the sole method of diagnosis.

3. **Blood Test:** A blood test can measure the levels of thyroid hormones and thyroid-stimulating hormone (TSH) in your body. While not a direct measure of iodine, abnormal levels of these hormones can indicate an iodine deficiency affecting thyroid function.

Interpreting Test Results:

- **Urine Test:** The World Health Organization (WHO) provides guidelines on urinary iodine concentrations. Levels below 100 micrograms/L indicate iodine deficiency, while levels above 100 micrograms/L are considered adequate.

- **Blood Test:** Elevated TSH levels, along with low levels of thyroid hormones (T4 and T3), can suggest an underactive thyroid (hypothyroidism) due to iodine deficiency.

If you suspect an iodine deficiency, it's crucial to consult with a healthcare provider. They can recommend the most appropriate tests and interpret the results accurately. Based on the findings, they may suggest dietary adjustments to include more iodine-rich foods or the use of supplements. Remember, while addressing iodine deficiency is essential, it's equally important to avoid excessive intake, which can lead to other health issues. Monitoring and adjusting iodine levels should always be done under professional guidance to ensure optimal health and well-being.

Chapter 2: Common Myths About Iodine

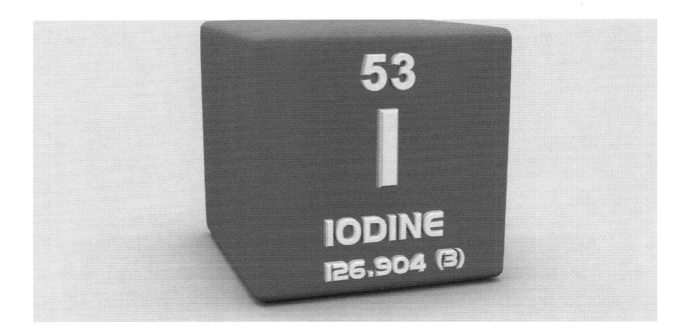

The Truth About Iodized Salt

Many individuals believe that simply using iodized salt in their daily cooking and consumption is enough to meet their iodine needs. However, this assumption falls short of the reality for several reasons. First, the amount of iodine in iodized salt can vary significantly. It's important to understand that during the processing of table salt, a small quantity of iodine is added to prevent deficiencies in the general population. Yet, the actual iodine content can diminish over time, especially if the salt is exposed to air and moisture, which can lead to a decrease in its potency.

Moreover, the modern diet and lifestyle have led to an increased consumption of processed foods, which rarely contain iodized salt. Instead, these foods are often made with non-iodized salt, thereby not contributing to the daily intake of iodine. Additionally, concerns about high blood pressure and heart disease have prompted many health-conscious individuals to reduce their overall salt intake, inadvertently affecting their iodine consumption as well.

Another critical aspect to consider is the bioavailability of iodine from iodized salt. Not all the iodine ingested through salt is fully absorbed by the body. Factors such as the presence of goitrogens in the diet – substances that interfere with iodine uptake – can further impede the efficient utilization of iodine from salt. Common goitrogens include certain types of vegetables, soy products, and even some grains and legumes.

Furthermore, the reliance on iodized salt alone overlooks the necessity for a varied diet rich in multiple sources of iodine. Foods such as seaweed, fish, dairy products, and eggs are naturally high in iodine and provide a more complex nutritional profile that can support thyroid health and overall well-being more effectively than iodized salt alone.

To ensure adequate iodine intake, it's advisable to incorporate a variety of iodine-rich foods into the diet. For individuals with specific health conditions or dietary restrictions that limit their iodine intake from food, consulting with a healthcare provider about supplementation may be a prudent approach. This ensures that the body receives the necessary amount of iodine for optimal thyroid function and metabolic health without relying solely on iodized salt, which may not provide sufficient levels of this crucial nutrient.

Debunking Iodophobia

The fear surrounding the use of iodine, often termed as "iodophobia," has its roots in misconceptions and a lack of understanding about this essential nutrient's role in our health. It's crucial to address these fears by examining the evidence and clarifying the benefits and safety of iodine supplementation when done correctly.

Firstly, the concern that iodine supplementation could lead to thyroid dysfunction is one of the primary fears. However, it's essential to understand that the thyroid gland requires iodine to produce thyroid hormones, which are critical for metabolism, growth, and development. The key is in the balance and ensuring that supplementation does not exceed recommended daily allowances unless under the guidance of a healthcare professional. Studies have shown that moderate iodine supplementation can support thyroid health, especially in populations where iodine deficiency is prevalent.

Another common fear is that iodine can be toxic and harmful to our health. This concern often stems from the misunderstanding of iodine's role and the difference between iodine and radioactive iodine, which is a completely different substance used in medical treatments. The toxicity of iodine is rare and usually occurs only when excessively high doses are consumed over a prolonged period. The tolerable upper intake level for adults, set by experts, is 1100 mcg per day, a threshold that is difficult to reach through a balanced diet and responsible supplementation.

The misconception that iodine intake can lead to autoimmune thyroid diseases also needs to be addressed. While it's true that in some cases, excessive iodine consumption has been linked to an increased risk of autoimmune thyroiditis, this risk is significantly lower than the risk posed by iodine deficiency. Proper iodine intake supports immune function and reduces inflammation, which can be beneficial in managing autoimmune conditions.

Lastly, the belief that we can get all the iodine we need from diet alone contributes to iodophobia, as it discourages supplementation. While it's true that foods such as seaweed, fish, and dairy are good sources of iodine, the reality is that many people do not consume enough of these foods regularly to meet their iodine needs. Soil depletion and modern agricultural practices have also reduced the iodine content in many foods, making it challenging for individuals to rely solely on diet for adequate iodine intake.

In conclusion, addressing iodophobia requires dispelling myths with facts and emphasizing the importance of iodine in supporting thyroid function, detoxification processes, and overall health. By understanding the role of iodine, recognizing the signs of deficiency, and following guidelines for safe supplementation, individuals can confidently incorporate this essential nutrient into their health regimen without fear.

Is Iodine Dangerous in Large Doses?

When discussing the safety of iodine, particularly in large doses, it's essential to distinguish between the necessity of this micronutrient for optimal health and the potential risks associated with excessive intake. Iodine plays a crucial role in thyroid function, metabolic regulation, and immune response. However, like many substances that benefit the body, there is a threshold beyond which iodine can become detrimental.

The body's requirement for iodine varies based on age, health status, and life stage. The Recommended Dietary Allowance (RDA) for adults is 150 micrograms (mcg) per day, with increased amounts recommended for pregnant and breastfeeding women due to the critical role iodine plays in fetal and neonatal neurological development. The Tolerable Upper Intake Level (UL) for iodine, established to prevent the risk of iodine-induced thyroid dysfunction, is set at 1100 mcg (1.1 mg) per day for adults. It's important to note that the UL is not a recommended level of intake but rather the maximum daily amount that is unlikely to cause adverse health effects in the general population.

Excessive iodine intake, particularly from supplements, can lead to various health issues, including but not limited to thyroid dysfunction. High levels of iodine can trigger either hypothyroidism or hyperthyroidism in susceptible individuals. In hypothyroidism, the thyroid gland becomes less efficient at producing thyroid hormones, leading to a slowdown in metabolic processes. Conversely, hyperthyroidism results from an overactive thyroid, which can accelerate metabolic functions to harmful levels. Both conditions are serious and require medical management.

Another concern with high iodine intake is the development of autoimmune thyroid diseases, such as Hashimoto's thyroiditis and Graves' disease. While the exact mechanism is not fully understood, it is believed that excessive iodine can initiate or exacerbate autoimmune responses in the thyroid gland in genetically predisposed individuals.

The risk of iodine toxicity, characterized by symptoms such as abdominal pain, nausea, vomiting, and even thyroid gland inflammation, increases with intake levels significantly above the UL. However, iodine toxicity is relatively rare and generally associated with doses many times higher than the UL or with exposure to iodine-containing medications or radiographic contrast agents rather than dietary intake.

For individuals considering iodine supplementation, particularly in doses that exceed the RDA, it is crucial to consult with a healthcare provider. This is especially important for those with existing thyroid conditions or autoimmune diseases, as they may be more vulnerable to the effects of excess iodine. A healthcare provider can offer guidance on appropriate supplementation based on individual health needs and can monitor for potential adverse effects.

Incorporating iodine into one's diet through food sources is generally considered safe and beneficial. Foods rich in iodine include seaweed, fish, dairy products, and eggs. These foods provide iodine in a form that the body can naturally regulate, reducing the risk of excessive intake.

For those using iodine supplements, it's advisable to stay informed about the iodine content of different products and to be mindful of the cumulative iodine intake from both dietary and supplemental sources. Awareness and moderation are key to harnessing the health benefits of iodine without risking adverse effects associated with excessive consumption.

Part 2: Practical Guide to Using Iodine

Chapter 3: Choosing and Using the Right Iodine

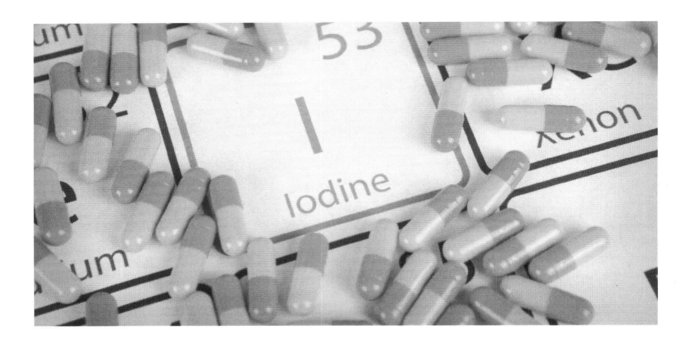

Types of Iodine Supplements

When considering supplementation to boost thyroid health, detoxify the body, enhance immunity, and increase energy levels, understanding the different types of iodine supplements available is crucial. Each form has unique characteristics and benefits, making it essential to choose the one that best suits your individual health needs.

Lugol's Solution is a time-tested supplement that has been used for over a century. It contains a specific ratio of potassium iodide (KI) and elemental iodine (I2). This combination is thought to offer a balanced approach to supplementation, as the body utilizes different forms of iodine for various physiological processes. Lugol's Solution is typically used in low doses and can be adjusted based on individual requirements. It's particularly favored for its ability to support thyroid function and its role in detoxification processes.

Nascent Iodine, often referred to as atomic iodine, is a form of iodine that is in a molecular state, which some believe is more easily absorbed by the body. This form is often recommended for those seeking to improve energy levels and cognitive function, as it is thought to be more bioavailable and therefore more effective at supporting the body's needs at a cellular level. Nascent iodine is usually found in a liquid form and can be taken in drops, making it easy to adjust dosages as needed.

Potassium Iodide (KI) is another common form of iodine supplementation, particularly known for its use in emergency situations to protect the thyroid gland from radioactive iodine exposure. However, it's also used for daily supplementation, especially in regions where iodine deficiency is common. Potassium iodide is absorbed by the thyroid gland and can help in maintaining healthy thyroid function. It is typically available in tablet form, making it a convenient option for many.

When selecting an iodine supplement, it's important to consider several factors, including your current health status, any existing thyroid conditions, and your specific health goals. For example, those with an underactive thyroid may find Lugol's Solution beneficial for its ability to support thyroid hormone production. On the other hand, individuals focusing on detoxification and cognitive function may prefer nascent iodine for its purported higher bioavailability.

Additionally, it's essential to start with a lower dosage and gradually increase as needed, paying close attention to how your body responds. Some individuals may experience detoxification symptoms as their body adjusts to the increased iodine intake. These symptoms are typically temporary but monitoring your body's reaction can help in adjusting your dosage to find the right balance for your needs.

Consulting with a healthcare provider who is knowledgeable about iodine supplementation can provide valuable guidance in selecting the right type of iodine for you. They can also recommend appropriate dosages based on your specific health situation and monitor your progress, adjusting the supplementation plan as necessary to ensure optimal health benefits.

Remember, while iodine is a critical nutrient for health, balance is key. Excessive intake can lead to adverse effects, just as deficiency can. Therefore, understanding the different forms of iodine supplements and their appropriate use is a vital step in safely incorporating this essential nutrient into your health regimen.

Which Iodine Is Right for You?

Selecting the appropriate form of iodine for your health regimen is a critical decision that hinges on various personal health factors and goals. The three primary forms of iodine supplementation—Lugol's Solution, Nascent Iodine, and Potassium Iodide—each offer distinct benefits and considerations. To make an informed choice, it's essential to evaluate your specific health needs, existing conditions, and objectives for supplementation.

Lugol's Solution, a blend of potassium iodide and elemental iodine, is well-suited for those seeking to support thyroid health due to its balanced composition. This form is particularly beneficial for individuals with an underactive thyroid or those looking to enhance their metabolic rate and energy levels. The dual presence of iodide and elemental iodine caters to the thyroid's needs, promoting the production of thyroid hormones. Starting with a low dose and adjusting based on your body's response and health improvements is advisable.

Nascent Iodine, recognized for its molecular form, is believed to be easily absorbed and utilized by the body. This option is optimal for individuals focusing on cellular energy, cognitive function, and detoxification. Its purported higher bioavailability means it may be more effective in supporting energy levels and brain health. Nascent iodine is typically administered in liquid form, allowing for flexible dosage adjustments. If you're aiming to boost mental clarity and detoxify, nascent iodine could be your go-to supplement.

Potassium Iodide (KI) is primarily known for its role in emergency situations to protect the thyroid from radioactive iodine. However, it's also beneficial for daily use, especially in areas where iodine deficiency is prevalent. This form is directly absorbed by the thyroid gland, supporting its function and health. Potassium iodide is a straightforward choice for those looking to maintain thyroid health without the additional benefits of elemental iodine. It's available in tablet form, offering convenience and ease of use.

When deciding which iodine is right for you, consider the following steps:

1. **Assess Your Health Status**: Evaluate your current thyroid function, energy levels, and any known deficiencies. Understanding your starting point helps in choosing the most beneficial form of iodine.

2. **Define Your Goals**: Are you looking to improve thyroid health, enhance cognitive function, or support detoxification? Your primary objective will guide your choice of iodine supplement.

3. **Consult a Healthcare Provider**: Before starting any new supplement, especially if you have existing health conditions or take other medications, seek advice from a healthcare professional. They can provide personalized recommendations based on your health status and goals.

4. **Start Low and Go Slow**: Begin with a lower dose of the chosen iodine form to monitor how your body responds. Adjust the dosage gradually, based on your body's reactions and health improvements.

5. **Monitor Your Progress**: Keep track of any changes in your symptoms or overall health. Adjustments to your supplementation may be necessary as your needs or health status changes.

By carefully considering these factors and steps, you can select the iodine supplement that aligns with your health needs and goals. Remember, the key to effective supplementation is not just the type of iodine you choose but also how well it matches your individual requirements and how you integrate it into a comprehensive health plan.

Iodine in Food Sources

Incorporating iodine-rich foods into your diet is a natural and effective way to support your thyroid health, enhance detoxification processes, boost your immune system, and increase your energy levels. The essential element plays a crucial role in the synthesis of thyroid hormones, which are pivotal for regulating metabolism, growth, and energy production. Despite its importance, many individuals may not achieve the recommended intake of iodine through diet alone, especially in regions where the soil is deficient in this nutrient. Here, we delve into various food sources that are abundant in iodine, offering a practical approach to enrich your diet.

Sea Vegetables: Seaweed stands out as the most potent source of iodine. Varieties such as kelp, nori, and wakame can significantly contribute to your daily intake. Just a single gram of dried seaweed can fulfill your iodine requirement for the day. Incorporating seaweed into soups, salads, or sushi is an excellent way to enjoy its benefits.

Fish and Shellfish: Seafood is another excellent source of iodine. Cod, shrimp, tuna, and scallops contain high levels of this mineral. Regular consumption of fish and shellfish can help maintain adequate iodine levels, supporting thyroid function and overall health.

Dairy Products: Milk, cheese, and yogurt are good sources of iodine, primarily because of the iodine supplements fed to cows and the use of iodine-containing disinfectants in dairy processing. Including dairy products in your diet can contribute to your iodine intake.

Eggs: Eggs are a versatile source of iodine, with the yolk containing the majority of the nutrient. They also provide a range of other essential vitamins and minerals, making them a valuable addition to a balanced diet.

Iodized Salt: While not a natural food source, iodized salt is a significant source of dietary iodine, especially in countries where iodine deficiency is common. A small amount can meet daily requirements; however, it's important to use it judiciously, considering the health implications of excessive sodium intake.

Prunes: A lesser-known source, prunes offer a modest amount of iodine. Consuming a few prunes daily can be a simple way to help reach your iodine intake goals, along with providing fiber and other nutrients.

Cranberries: This tart fruit is another natural source of iodine. Fresh cranberries or a small serving of cranberry juice can contribute to your daily iodine intake while offering antioxidant benefits.

To effectively incorporate these iodine-rich foods into your diet, consider the following strategies:

- Start your day with a breakfast that includes dairy products or eggs, providing a morning boost of iodine.
- Add seaweed to your meals several times a week, whether in salads, soups, or as a snack.
- Include fish or shellfish in your diet 2-3 times per week to ensure a steady intake of iodine.
- Use iodized salt in moderation to season your meals.
- Snack on prunes or include cranberries in your diet for an additional source of iodine.

By diversifying your food sources and incorporating these iodine-rich options into your daily meals, you can naturally support your thyroid health and overall well-being. Remember, while dietary sources of iodine are essential, it's crucial to monitor your intake and consult with a healthcare provider to ensure you're meeting your body's needs without exceeding the recommended limits.

Chapter 4: Safely Incorporating Iodine

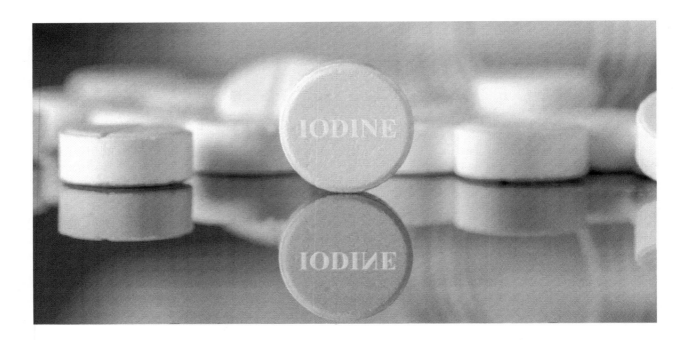

Step-by-Step Dosage Guidelines

When embarking on a regimen involving iodine supplementation, it's crucial to adhere to precise dosage guidelines to optimize thyroid health, detoxification processes, and immune function while minimizing the risk of adverse effects. The following step-by-step instructions are designed to cater to both beginners and advanced users, ensuring a tailored approach to meet individual health objectives and current iodine status.

Beginners:

1. **Initial Assessment**: Before starting supplementation, consult with a healthcare provider to assess your current iodine levels through appropriate testing. This step is vital to determine your starting point.

2. **Low-Dose Introduction**: Begin with a low dose of iodine, typically around 150-300 micrograms (mcg) per day. This dosage aligns with the Recommended Dietary Allowance (RDA) and serves as a cautious introduction to supplementation.

3. **Gradual Increase**: If well-tolerated, and under the guidance of your healthcare provider, gradually increase the dosage every two to three weeks. Pay attention to your body's response to each adjustment.

4. **Monitoring**: Keep a log of any changes in symptoms, energy levels, or side effects. Regular follow-up tests are recommended to monitor iodine levels and thyroid function.

Advanced Users:

1. **Medical Supervision**: For those considering higher doses, especially doses exceeding 1,200 mcg (1.2 mg) per day, medical supervision is imperative. Higher intakes are typically explored for specific health conditions and should not be initiated without professional guidance.

2. **Incremental Adjustments**: Increase the dosage in small increments, allowing sufficient time for the body to adjust. This approach helps identify the optimal dose that supports health without inducing hyperthyroidism or other adverse effects.

3. **Detoxification Support**: At higher dosages, iodine may mobilize stored toxins such as bromide and fluoride. Incorporating a salt loading protocol and ensuring adequate hydration can assist in flushing these toxins from the body.

4. **Synergistic Nutrients**: Supplementing with selenium (200 mcg daily), magnesium, and vitamin C can support thyroid function and antioxidant defenses, enhancing the benefits of iodine and mitigating potential side effects.

General Recommendations:

- **Iodine Sources**: While supplements provide a controlled iodine intake, incorporating natural sources like seaweed, fish, and dairy can offer additional benefits. Balance is key, as dietary sources contribute to overall iodine intake.

- **Listen to Your Body**: Individual responses to iodine supplementation can vary widely. Symptoms such as palpitations, anxiety, or changes in thyroid function tests may indicate the need to adjust the dosage.

- **Adaptation Period**: Some individuals may experience detoxification symptoms as the body adjusts to increased iodine levels. These symptoms typically resolve with time and proper supportive measures.

Adhering to these guidelines allows for a personalized and safe approach to iodine supplementation, supporting thyroid health and overall well-being. Regular consultation with healthcare professionals ensures that the supplementation strategy remains aligned with your health status and goals.

Adapting Iodine for Thyroid, Detox, and Energy

Tailoring iodine supplementation to individual needs is crucial for optimizing thyroid function, enhancing detoxification, and boosting energy levels. Each person's body responds differently to iodine, influenced by factors like baseline thyroid health, exposure to environmental toxins, and overall energy requirements. Therefore, understanding how to adjust iodine intake for specific health goals is essential.

Thyroid Health: For individuals dealing with hypothyroidism or general thyroid underactivity, the focus should be on supporting the thyroid gland's ability to produce hormones. Starting with a modest dose of iodine, such as 150-300 micrograms daily, can be beneficial. If the body tolerates this well, and under the guidance of a healthcare provider, the amount may be gradually increased. It's important to monitor thyroid function tests regularly to ensure that the supplementation is supporting, rather than overwhelming, the thyroid gland. In cases of autoimmune thyroid conditions like Hashimoto's thyroiditis, careful monitoring is even more critical, as excessive iodine can sometimes exacerbate these conditions.

Detoxification: For those primarily interested in iodine's detoxifying benefits, particularly for flushing out heavy metals and halides like fluoride and bromide, a slightly different approach may be warranted. After establishing tolerance to a baseline dose, individuals may consider a moderate increase in iodine intake, accompanied by the salt loading protocol to facilitate toxin removal. This method involves consuming a larger amount of salt and water to encourage the excretion of bromide and fluoride through urine. It's advisable to include antioxidants like selenium, vitamin C, and magnesium to support the body during detoxification. Monitoring for detox symptoms is crucial, and adjustments should be made based on the body's responses.

Energy Restoration: For those seeking to boost energy and metabolism, iodine can play a pivotal role by enhancing mitochondrial efficiency—the energy powerhouses of the cell. In this context, ensuring adequate iodine intake to support thyroid function is the first step, as the thyroid hormones directly influence metabolic rate and energy levels. Starting with the recommended dietary allowance and adjusting based on energy levels and metabolic markers can help identify the optimal dose for energy enhancement. Incorporating a balanced diet rich in iodine sources and other nutrients that support energy metabolism, such as B vitamins and iron, is also beneficial.

In all cases, it's vital to listen to your body and adjust supplementation based on personal health outcomes. Some individuals may experience signs of over-supplementation, such as jitteriness, increased heart rate, or sleep disturbances, indicating the need to reassess iodine intake. Regular follow-ups with a healthcare provider can help navigate these adjustments and ensure that iodine supplementation is contributing positively to health without causing adverse effects.

Supporting iodine intake with a diet rich in natural sources of the mineral and other synergistic nutrients can enhance the benefits of supplementation. Whether the goal is to support thyroid health, enhance detoxification, or boost energy levels, a personalized approach to iodine supplementation can help achieve these health objectives effectively.

Avoiding Overuse and Side Effects

To mitigate the risk of overuse and the potential side effects associated with iodine supplementation, it is essential to approach this aspect of your health regimen with informed caution and precision. The key to avoiding adverse reactions lies in understanding the balance between beneficial and excessive intake, recognizing signs of overuse, and implementing strategies to prevent or address side effects. Here are actionable steps and considerations to ensure a safe and effective use of iodine for health optimization:

1. **Start with the Minimum Effective Dose**: Begin your supplementation with the lowest dose that has been shown to produce health benefits. For many, this might mean adhering closely to the Recommended Dietary Allowance (RDA) before gradually increasing the amount based on individual needs and under professional guidance.

2. **Monitor Your Response**: Pay close attention to how your body reacts to the supplementation. Common signs of excessive iodine intake include changes in thyroid function, such as hypothyroidism or hyperthyroidism, as well as more immediate symptoms like a metallic taste in the mouth, mouth sores, or gastrointestinal discomfort. Documenting these reactions can help in adjusting dosages promptly and appropriately.

3. **Regular Testing**: Undergoing periodic thyroid function tests and iodine level assessments can provide concrete data on how your supplementation regimen affects your health. This practice is crucial for fine-tuning your intake and avoiding both deficiency and excess.

4. **Incorporate Supporting Nutrients**: Ensuring adequate intake of selenium, zinc, and magnesium can support thyroid health and mitigate potential side effects of iodine supplementation. These minerals work synergistically with iodine, promoting optimal thyroid function and detoxification processes.

5. **Stay Hydrated**: Adequate hydration supports the body's natural detoxification pathways, including the elimination of excess iodine. Drinking sufficient water throughout the day can help minimize the risk of iodine-related side effects.

6. **Dietary Balance**: While supplements can be a powerful tool for addressing iodine deficiency, obtaining this nutrient from natural food sources where possible can offer a more balanced approach. Foods like seaweed, fish, and dairy provide iodine in conjunction with other beneficial nutrients, potentially reducing the risk of over-supplementation.

7. **Consult Healthcare Professionals**: Before starting, adjusting, or stopping iodine supplementation, consult with a healthcare provider. This is especially important for

individuals with pre-existing thyroid conditions, pregnant or breastfeeding women, and those on medication that could interact with iodine.

8. **Adjustment Period**: Recognize that some symptoms might arise as the body adjusts to increased iodine levels, particularly if you are correcting a deficiency. These symptoms are often temporary and should be monitored closely. If they persist or worsen, it may indicate the need for adjustment in your supplementation protocol.

9. **Be Cautious with High Doses**: High-dose iodine supplementation should only be considered under medical supervision for specific health conditions. If advised to pursue such a regimen, ensure that it is closely monitored for efficacy and safety.

10. **Listen to Your Body**: Ultimately, each individual's response to iodine will vary. Being attuned to the subtle cues your body provides can guide you in making the necessary adjustments to your supplementation strategy, ensuring that you derive the maximum benefit without adverse effects.

By adhering to these guidelines, individuals can safely incorporate iodine into their health regimen, leveraging its numerous benefits while minimizing the risk of overuse and side effects. Regular consultation with healthcare professionals and a mindful approach to supplementation are paramount in navigating this aspect of your wellness journey.

Chapter 5: Supporting Iodine with Nutrients

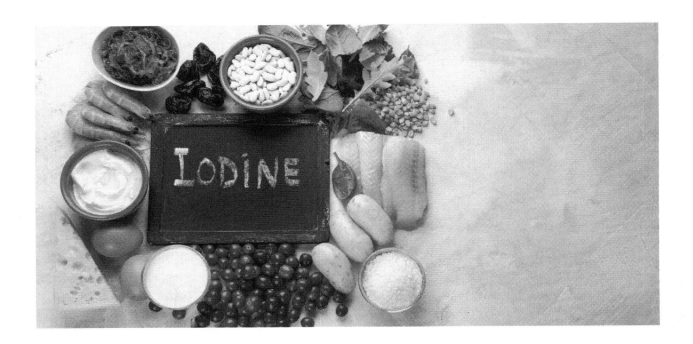

The Iodine-Selenium Connection

The synergy between iodine and selenium is a critical aspect of thyroid health and overall well-being. Both elements play pivotal roles in the proper functioning of the thyroid gland, and their interaction enhances the body's ability to utilize iodine effectively. Selenium, a trace element, is essential for the conversion of thyroid hormone T4 (thyroxine) into its active form, T3 (triiodothyronine). This conversion process is crucial for regulating metabolism, energy production, and maintaining homeostasis.

Selenium's Role in Antioxidant Protection: Selenium acts as a cofactor for glutathione peroxidase, an enzyme that protects the thyroid gland from oxidative damage caused by hydrogen peroxide, a byproduct of thyroid hormone production. Adequate selenium intake ensures the integrity of the thyroid gland and supports the body's antioxidant defenses, reducing the risk of thyroid dysfunction.

Iodine and Selenium Balance: Maintaining a balance between iodine and selenium is essential for thyroid health. An excess of iodine without sufficient selenium can lead to an increased risk of developing autoimmune thyroid diseases, such as Hashimoto's thyroiditis. Conversely, adequate selenium levels can mitigate the potential adverse effects of excessive iodine intake on the thyroid gland.

Recommended Selenium Intake: For adults, the recommended dietary allowance (RDA) for selenium is 55 micrograms (mcg) per day. Sources of selenium include Brazil nuts, seafood, organ meats, and cereals. Incorporating these foods into your diet can help achieve the necessary selenium intake to support thyroid function and enhance the efficacy of iodine supplementation.

Strategies for Optimizing Iodine and Selenium Intake:

1. **Diversify Your Diet:** Include a variety of selenium-rich foods in your diet to ensure adequate intake. Just one or two Brazil nuts a day can provide the RDA for selenium. Adding seafood, such as tuna, shrimp, and salmon, can also contribute to both iodine and selenium intake.

2. **Consider Supplementation:** If dietary sources are insufficient or if you have specific health conditions that increase your need for selenium or iodine, consider supplementation under the guidance of a healthcare provider. It's important to monitor levels regularly to avoid imbalances.

3. **Monitor Thyroid Function:** Regularly check your thyroid function and levels of thyroid hormones, especially if you are supplementing with iodine and selenium. This will help in adjusting dosages to maintain optimal thyroid health.

4. **Be Mindful of Interactions:** Some compounds, such as certain minerals and medications, can interfere with the absorption and utilization of iodine and selenium. Discuss with your healthcare provider to identify any potential interactions and adjust your supplementation strategy accordingly.

5. **Adjust Intake Based on Needs:** Factors such as age, pregnancy, lactation, and health conditions can affect your iodine and selenium requirements. Tailor your intake to your specific needs, aiming for a balanced approach that supports thyroid health without causing imbalances.

Incorporating these strategies into your health regimen can optimize the benefits of iodine and selenium for thyroid function and overall wellness. By understanding the intricate relationship between these two essential nutrients, you can take proactive steps to support your thyroid health and enhance your body's detoxification processes, immunity, and energy levels.

Other Key Nutrients: Magnesium, Zinc, Vitamin D

Magnesium, zinc, and vitamin D are pivotal in enhancing the benefits of iodine, each playing a unique role in supporting thyroid health and overall well-being. Understanding how these nutrients work in tandem with iodine can empower individuals to optimize their health strategies effectively.

Magnesium is essential for the activation of thyroid hormones. Without adequate magnesium levels, the thyroid cannot operate efficiently, leading to potential issues with metabolism and energy production. Magnesium also aids in the detoxification processes that are crucial for removing harmful substances from the body. Incorporating foods rich in magnesium, such as leafy greens, nuts, seeds, and whole grains, or considering a high-quality magnesium supplement, can support iodine in maintaining thyroid health and enhancing detoxification.

Zinc plays a critical role in thyroid hormone synthesis and metabolism. It is involved in converting the inactive thyroid hormone (T4) into its active form (T3), a process essential for metabolic health. Zinc deficiency has been linked to reduced thyroid function and hypothyroidism. To ensure adequate zinc levels, include zinc-rich foods like oysters, beef, pumpkin seeds, and lentils in your diet or consider a zinc supplement after consulting with a healthcare provider.

Vitamin D is another nutrient that supports thyroid function and immune health. It has been shown to influence the production and regulation of thyroid hormones. Vitamin D deficiency is common in individuals with autoimmune thyroid disorders, such as Hashimoto's thyroiditis. Safe sun exposure, vitamin D-rich foods like fatty fish and fortified products, and supplementation can help maintain optimal levels of this nutrient, thereby supporting thyroid health and immune function.

For individuals looking to support their thyroid health and enhance the detoxification benefits of iodine, paying attention to the intake of magnesium, zinc, and vitamin D is crucial. Assessing dietary sources and considering supplementation if necessary, under the guidance of a healthcare professional, can provide a comprehensive approach to optimizing the synergistic effects of these nutrients with iodine.

Salt Loading for Bromide Detox

The technique of salt loading is a pivotal strategy for facilitating the detoxification of bromide from the body. Bromide, a halide like iodine, competes with iodine for absorption and utilization in the thyroid gland and other tissues. When individuals increase their iodine intake, either through diet or supplementation, the body begins to displace bromide and other toxic halides, which can lead to an array of detoxification symptoms. Salt loading can help expedite the excretion of these displaced bromides, mitigating the discomfort associated with detoxification.

To effectively implement salt loading for bromide detox, one must understand the process and follow a structured approach. The method involves ingesting a solution of high-quality, unrefined salt dissolved in water. The salt solution works by encouraging the kidneys to excrete bromide through urine, thus aiding in the detoxification process. Here is a step-by-step guide to salt loading:

1. **Prepare the Salt Solution**: Dissolve half a teaspoon of unrefined sea salt or Himalayan pink salt in 8 ounces (about 240 milliliters) of warm water. It's crucial to use unrefined salt because it contains a variety of minerals that refined table salt lacks.

2. **Consume the Salt Solution**: Drink the salt solution. It's best to do this in the morning, as it can increase energy levels and may interfere with sleep if taken too late in the day.

3. **Follow with Additional Water**: After drinking the salt solution, follow it with an additional 12-16 ounces (about 355-475 milliliters) of filtered water within the next 30 minutes to an hour. This helps to ensure that the kidneys can efficiently flush out the bromide.

4. **Monitor Your Response**: Pay attention to how your body responds to the salt loading protocol. Some individuals may experience increased urination, which is a sign that the body is excreting bromide. If you experience bloating or swelling, it may indicate that the salt concentration is too high for your body, and you should adjust the dosage accordingly.

5. **Adjust as Needed**: If you do not notice an improvement in detoxification symptoms or if you experience adverse effects, you may need to adjust the amount of salt or the frequency of the protocol. Some individuals may require less salt, while others may benefit from repeating the salt loading process two to three times a day, depending on the severity of their symptoms and their overall health status.

6. **Support with Hydration and Nutrition**: Enhance the effectiveness of the salt loading protocol by maintaining adequate hydration throughout the day and consuming a nutrient-dense diet. Foods rich in antioxidants, vitamins, and minerals support the body's natural detoxification pathways and can help mitigate detox symptoms.

It's important to note that while salt loading can be an effective method for supporting bromide detoxification, it's not suitable for everyone. Individuals with hypertension, kidney disease, or any condition that requires sodium restriction should consult with a healthcare professional before attempting the salt loading protocol. Additionally, integrating other supportive practices, such as consuming iodine-rich foods and supplements, ensuring adequate intake of selenium, magnesium, and vitamin C, and engaging in regular exercise, can further aid in the detoxification process and support overall thyroid health and well-being.

PART 3: Healing with Iodine

Chapter 6: Iodine and Thyroid Health

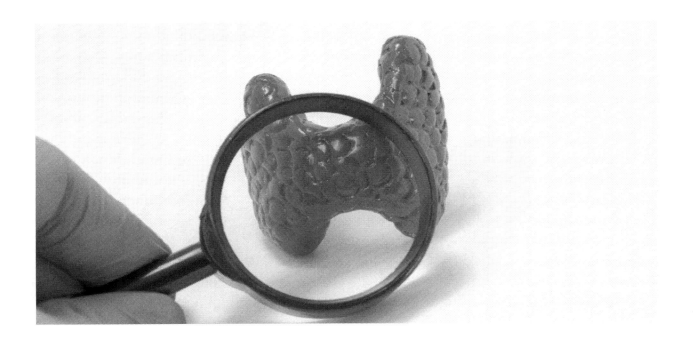

Healing Hypothyroidism

Hypothyroidism, a condition where the thyroid gland is underactive, can lead to a myriad of health issues, including fatigue, weight gain, and depression. The thyroid gland requires iodine to produce thyroid hormones, which are critical for regulating metabolism, energy levels, and overall bodily functions. An adequate intake of this mineral can support the thyroid in its hormone production, naturally aiding in the management and potential healing of hypothyroidism.

Iodine's Role in Thyroid Hormone Production: The thyroid gland synthesizes two main hormones, thyroxine (T4) and triiodothyronine (T3), both of which require iodine. An insufficient amount of iodine can lead to decreased production of these hormones, contributing to hypothyroid symptoms. Ensuring an adequate intake of iodine can help support the thyroid gland's needs for hormone production, thus addressing one of the root causes of hypothyroidism.

Increasing Iodine Intake: For individuals with hypothyroidism, increasing iodine intake through diet or supplementation can be a crucial step. Foods rich in iodine include seaweed, dairy products, eggs, and fish. For some, iodine supplements may be necessary to reach the recommended daily intake. However, it's important to approach supplementation with caution, as excessive iodine can also lead to thyroid issues. Consulting with a healthcare provider to determine the appropriate dosage is essential.

Monitoring Iodine Levels: Regular monitoring of iodine levels through urinary iodine concentration tests can provide valuable insights into whether an individual is getting enough iodine or potentially over-supplementing. This monitoring can help in adjusting iodine intake to maintain optimal thyroid function.

Addressing Autoimmune Thyroid Disorders: In cases of autoimmune thyroid disorders like Hashimoto's thyroiditis, where the body's immune system attacks the thyroid gland, managing iodine intake becomes more complex. While iodine is crucial for thyroid health, its role in autoimmune thyroid conditions is nuanced, and excessive intake may exacerbate the condition. Working closely with a healthcare provider to tailor iodine intake is crucial in these scenarios.

Supporting Nutrients: Alongside iodine, other nutrients play supportive roles in thyroid health. Selenium, for example, is vital for the conversion of T4 to the more active T3 hormone and can protect the thyroid gland from oxidative stress. Similarly, zinc and vitamin D are important for thyroid function and overall immune health. Ensuring a balanced intake of these nutrients can enhance the benefits of iodine for individuals with hypothyroidism.

Lifestyle Considerations: Beyond dietary adjustments, lifestyle factors such as stress management, regular exercise, and avoiding exposure to toxins can also support thyroid health. These practices, combined with adequate iodine intake, create a holistic approach to managing hypothyroidism.

Personalized Approach: Each individual's needs and response to iodine supplementation can vary, making a personalized approach essential. Factors such as the severity of hypothyroidism, presence of autoimmune thyroid disorders, and overall health status should guide iodine and nutrient intake strategies.

Incorporating these strategies can support the natural healing process of hypothyroidism by ensuring the thyroid gland has the necessary iodine for hormone production. It's a delicate balance that requires careful consideration and, often, professional guidance to navigate effectively.

Autoimmune Thyroid Disorders

Autoimmune thyroid disorders such as Hashimoto's thyroiditis and Graves' disease present unique challenges in the management of thyroid health. These conditions, where the immune system mistakenly attacks the thyroid gland, require a nuanced approach to iodine supplementation. In Hashimoto's, the immune system targets the thyroid, leading to potential hypothyroidism, whereas Graves' disease often results in hyperthyroidism due to the production of antibodies that stimulate the thyroid to produce too much hormone.

Iodine's Role in Autoimmune Thyroid Disorders: The element plays a critical role in thyroid hormone production. However, its impact on autoimmune thyroid conditions is complex. For some, adequate iodine intake can support thyroid function, but for others, especially those with Hashimoto's, excessive intake might exacerbate the condition. The key is finding a balance that supports thyroid health without triggering an immune response.

Strategies for Managing Iodine Intake:

1. **Start with Testing**: Before adjusting iodine intake, it's crucial to assess current iodine levels through urinary iodine concentration tests. This initial step helps tailor the approach to individual needs.

2. **Gradual Supplementation**: For those with diagnosed autoimmune thyroid disorders, gradually introducing iodine, if deemed necessary by healthcare providers, can help monitor the body's response. This cautious approach allows for adjustments based on symptoms and test results.

3. **Monitor Thyroid Function**: Regular monitoring of thyroid function tests, including TSH, Free T4, and Free T3, alongside thyroid antibody levels, can provide insights into how well the thyroid is responding to iodine supplementation and whether adjustments are needed.

4. **Incorporate Selenium**: Selenium supplementation may benefit individuals with autoimmune thyroid conditions by reducing thyroid antibody levels. This nutrient supports efficient thyroid hormone synthesis and metabolism and may offer protective effects against oxidative stress within the thyroid gland.

5. **Lifestyle Modifications**: Emphasizing a diet rich in anti-inflammatory foods, managing stress through techniques such as yoga or meditation, and avoiding known dietary triggers can complement iodine management strategies. These lifestyle factors contribute to overall immune system health, potentially reducing autoimmune activity against the thyroid.

6. **Collaborate with Healthcare Providers**: Given the complexity of autoimmune thyroid disorders, working closely with healthcare providers is essential. This collaboration ensures that iodine intake, whether through diet or supplementation, is appropriately managed to support thyroid health without aggravating the autoimmune process.

Understanding the Impact of Iodine on Autoimmune Thyroid Disorders: It's important to recognize that the relationship between iodine and autoimmune thyroid diseases is influenced by several factors, including genetic predisposition, environmental triggers, and individual nutritional status. While iodine is a fundamental nutrient for thyroid health, its role in autoimmune conditions underscores the importance of a personalized approach. Each individual's experience with Hashimoto's or Graves' disease is unique, necessitating a tailored strategy that considers the delicate balance between providing sufficient iodine for thyroid hormone production and minimizing the risk of immune system activation.

For those navigating the complexities of autoimmune thyroid disorders, the goal is to support thyroid function and immune health through careful management of iodine intake, complemented by broader nutritional and lifestyle strategies. This comprehensive approach aims to enhance quality of life and promote optimal thyroid health amidst the challenges posed by autoimmune conditions.

Iodine's Role in Thyroid Cancer Prevention

The significance of iodine in the prevention of thyroid cancer cannot be overstated. Thyroid cancer, characterized by the abnormal growth of cells in the thyroid gland, has been linked to various risk factors, including iodine deficiency. The thyroid gland uses iodine to produce thyroid hormones, which are crucial for regulating metabolism, growth, and development. When the body lacks sufficient iodine, the thyroid gland can undergo changes that may increase the risk of developing cancerous cells.

Iodine's Protective Mechanism: Iodine contributes to the normal functioning of the thyroid gland, helping to prevent the development of thyroid nodules, which can be precursors to cancer. It is involved in the synthesis of thyroid hormones, and adequate levels of iodine help ensure the thyroid gland does not have to overwork, a condition that can lead to the formation of goiters and, potentially, to the development of thyroid cancer.

Research Findings: Studies have shown that populations in regions with iodine-deficient diets have a higher incidence of goiter and, subsequently, a higher risk of thyroid cancer. Supplementation of iodine in these populations has been associated with a decrease in the incidence of goiter and possibly a reduced risk of thyroid cancer. This correlation underscores the importance of maintaining adequate iodine levels for thyroid health and cancer prevention.

Recommended Iodine Intake: The recommended dietary allowance (RDA) for iodine varies by age, gender, and life stage, with adults generally advised to consume 150 micrograms per day. Pregnant and lactating women have higher requirements due to the increased need for iodine during these periods. It is crucial to consult with a healthcare provider to determine the appropriate iodine intake for your specific needs, especially if you have existing thyroid conditions or are at risk for thyroid cancer.

Sources of Iodine: Incorporating iodine-rich foods into your diet is a practical approach to ensuring adequate intake. Seafood, dairy products, eggs, and iodized salt are excellent sources of iodine. For individuals who may not get enough iodine from their diet alone, iodine supplements can be an effective alternative. However, it is essential to approach supplementation with caution, as excessive iodine intake can also lead to thyroid dysfunction.

Monitoring Iodine Levels: Regular monitoring of iodine levels can help identify deficiencies or excesses that could impact thyroid health. Urinary iodine concentration tests offer a non-invasive method to assess iodine status. Additionally, thyroid function tests can provide insights into how well the thyroid gland is working and whether adjustments to iodine intake may be necessary.

Combining Iodine with Other Nutrients: For optimal thyroid health and cancer prevention, iodine should not be considered in isolation. Selenium, zinc, and vitamin D also play vital roles in supporting thyroid function and immune health. A balanced intake of these nutrients, alongside iodine, can provide a comprehensive approach to maintaining thyroid health and reducing the risk of thyroid cancer.

Personalized Approach: Given the variability in iodine needs and the potential risks associated with both deficiency and excess, a personalized approach to iodine supplementation is advised. Factors such as dietary habits, health status, and risk factors for thyroid disease should guide decisions regarding iodine intake. Consulting with healthcare professionals who can provide tailored advice based on your individual needs and health status is essential.

In summary, the role of iodine in preventing thyroid cancer highlights the broader importance of micronutrients in maintaining health and preventing disease. By ensuring adequate iodine intake through diet or supplements, monitoring iodine levels, and considering the synergistic effects of other nutrients, individuals can take proactive steps towards reducing their risk of thyroid cancer and supporting overall thyroid health.

Chapter 7: Detoxing Your Body with Iodine

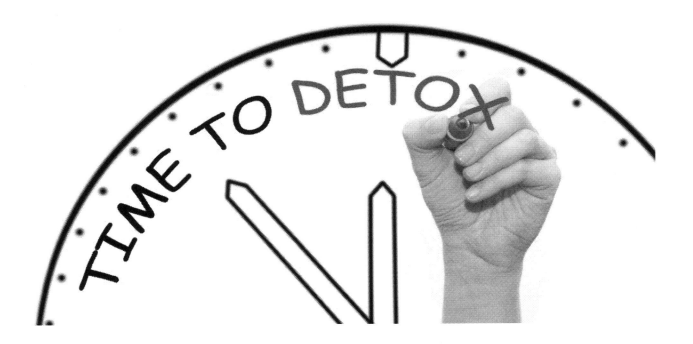

Detoxing Heavy Metals with Iodine

Heavy metals like mercury and lead pose significant health risks, including neurological damage and impaired organ function. Iodine plays a crucial role in the body's detoxification process, aiding in the removal of these toxic substances. When iodine levels are optimal, the thyroid functions efficiently, enhancing metabolic processes that facilitate the elimination of heavy metals.

The mechanism by which iodine assists in detoxifying heavy metals involves its ability to support the thyroid gland. A healthy thyroid gland produces hormones that regulate metabolism, which is vital for detoxification. These hormones stimulate the liver, kidneys, and intestines, organs responsible for filtering and excreting toxins.

Furthermore, iodine itself can act as a chelating agent. This means it can bind to heavy metals, making them more water-soluble and easier for the body to excrete. This process is particularly important for metals like mercury and lead, which are otherwise difficult for the body to eliminate.

Incorporating iodine into your detox plan requires careful consideration of dosage and form. For detox purposes, a higher intake of iodine may be necessary, but it's crucial to increase the dosage gradually to monitor the body's response and avoid potential side effects. Forms of iodine such as Lugol's solution or nascent iodine are often recommended for their efficacy and bioavailability.

Supporting iodine intake with a diet rich in selenium, zinc, and vitamin C can enhance the detoxification process. Selenium, for example, works synergistically with iodine to support thyroid function and can also help protect against oxidative damage caused by heavy metals.

To effectively detox heavy metals with iodine, consider the following steps:
1. Start with a baseline iodine supplementation, gradually increasing the dose while monitoring for any adverse reactions.
2. Incorporate foods high in natural iodine, such as seaweed, fish, and dairy, into your diet.
3. Supplement with selenium, zinc, and vitamin C to support the detox process and protect against oxidative stress.
4. Stay hydrated and consider practices like salt water flushes or baths to aid in the excretion of bound toxins.
5. Regularly consult with a healthcare provider to monitor heavy metal levels and adjust the detox plan as necessary.

It's important to approach iodine supplementation with caution, especially in the context of detoxification. The body's response to increased iodine intake can vary, and in some cases, it may initially exacerbate symptoms as toxins are mobilized for excretion. Regular monitoring and adjustment of the detox protocol are essential to safely and effectively reduce heavy metal levels in the body.

Fluoride and Bromide Detox

Fluoride and bromide are common elements found in our environment, but their accumulation in the body can disrupt thyroid function and overall health. These halides compete with iodine for absorption and utilization in the thyroid gland, leading to iodine deficiency and a host of related health issues. Detoxifying your body of these substances is a critical step toward restoring balance and enhancing your well-being.

Fluoride, primarily sourced from drinking water, dental products, and certain medications, can be challenging to avoid. To reduce fluoride intake, consider installing a water filtration system that specifically removes fluoride. Reverse osmosis filters are particularly effective. Additionally, opt for fluoride-free toothpaste and mouth rinses. Be mindful of foods and beverages prepared with fluoridated water, as these can also contribute to your fluoride levels.

Bromide is found in commercial baked goods, some soft drinks, and certain medications and pesticides. To minimize exposure, choose organic produce whenever possible and avoid processed foods, especially those containing brominated vegetable oil (BVO). Reading labels can help you steer clear of products with bromide-containing ingredients.

To facilitate the detoxification of fluoride and bromide, increasing your iodine intake can be beneficial. Iodine competes with these halides for absorption, helping to flush them out of your system. However, it's essential to approach iodine supplementation with care, starting with a low dose and gradually increasing it to avoid potential side effects. Consulting with a healthcare provider knowledgeable about iodine therapy is advisable to tailor the approach to your specific needs.

In addition to iodine supplementation, supporting your detox pathways is crucial. Ensure adequate hydration to help flush toxins from your body. A diet rich in antioxidants, such as fruits and vegetables, can protect against oxidative stress during detoxification. Foods high in selenium, such as Brazil nuts, sunflower seeds, and fish, can aid in the excretion of halides by supporting thyroid function and enhancing iodine's effectiveness.

Engaging in regular exercise and sweating through activities like sauna sessions can also accelerate the removal of toxins, including fluoride and bromide. Epsom salt baths may aid in detoxification by providing magnesium, which supports detox pathways and overall health.

Remember, detoxing from fluoride and bromide is a gradual process. It requires patience, consistency, and a holistic approach to diet and lifestyle. Monitoring your progress with the guidance of a healthcare professional can help you adjust your strategy as needed, ensuring a safe and effective detox journey.

Creating a Detox Plan

To create an effective detox plan using iodine, it's essential to approach the process with a structured and informed strategy. This plan is designed to gradually increase iodine intake, support the body's natural detoxification pathways, and minimize potential detox symptoms. Here's how to get started:

1. **Assess Your Current Health Status**: Before adding iodine to your regimen, evaluate your current health, focusing on thyroid function and potential toxic exposures. Consulting with a healthcare professional can provide insights into your specific needs and any precautions you should take.

2. **Begin with a Low Dose**: Start with a low dose of iodine, such as 150-300 micrograms daily, to gently introduce it to your system. This dosage can help acclimate your body and reduce the risk of detox symptoms.

3. **Gradually Increase the Dose**: Depending on your tolerance and health goals, gradually increase the dose over weeks or months. A common target for detox purposes is between 12.5 mg and 50 mg daily, but this should be done under professional guidance.

4. **Incorporate Supporting Nutrients**: Enhance iodine's effectiveness and support detoxification by including nutrients such as selenium, vitamin C, magnesium, and zinc

in your diet or as supplements. These nutrients work synergistically with iodine and can help mitigate detox reactions.

5. **Stay Hydrated**: Adequate hydration is crucial during detoxification. Aim for at least 8-10 glasses of filtered water daily to help flush toxins from your body.

6. **Optimize Your Diet**: Focus on a nutrient-dense diet rich in antioxidants, fiber, and clean protein sources. Foods like leafy greens, berries, nuts, and seeds can support detox pathways and overall health.

7. **Monitor Your Response**: Pay close attention to how your body responds to the increased iodine intake. Symptoms such as fatigue, headaches, or skin reactions can indicate that your body is detoxifying. Adjust your plan as needed, reducing the dose temporarily if symptoms become uncomfortable.

8. **Consider Detox Aids**: Techniques such as dry brushing, sauna sessions, or Epsom salt baths can support the detox process by stimulating circulation and promoting the elimination of toxins through the skin.

9. **Regular Testing**: Work with your healthcare provider to monitor your iodine levels, thyroid function, and heavy metal levels throughout the detox process. This data can guide adjustments to your plan and ensure you're detoxifying safely.

10. **Listen to Your Body**: Everyone's detox journey is unique. If you experience adverse effects or if something doesn't feel right, it's crucial to listen to your body and adjust your approach accordingly. Sometimes, slowing down is the best way to achieve long-term success.

By following these steps, you can create a personalized iodine detox plan that supports your health goals while minimizing discomfort. Remember, the key to a successful detox is patience, consistency, and a willingness to adjust your approach based on your body's signals.

Chapter 8: Boosting Immunity and Energy

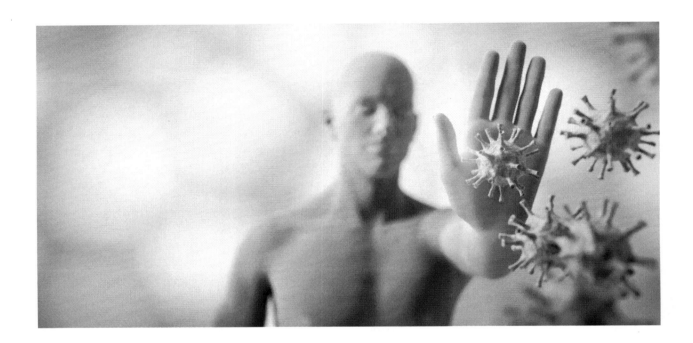

Strengthening Your Immune System

In bolstering the immune system, the role of iodine is pivotal yet often underestimated. This trace element is essential for the production of thyroid hormones, which in turn play a crucial role in regulating the immune response. A well-functioning thyroid gland ensures that the body's defense mechanisms operate efficiently, ready to fend off infections and combat chronic diseases.

Iodine's Impact on Immune Cells: The body's immune system comprises various types of cells designed to detect and destroy pathogens. Iodine directly influences the activity of these cells, enhancing their responsiveness to invaders. For instance, T-cells, which are vital for the immune response, rely on thyroid hormones to function optimally. Adequate iodine levels ensure that these hormones are produced in the right amounts, thus keeping the T-cells alert and active.

Regulation of Inflammation: Inflammation is the body's natural response to infection or injury, but chronic inflammation can lead to numerous health issues. Iodine plays a role in modulating the body's inflammatory responses, ensuring they are not excessive and do not cause unnecessary damage. This regulation helps prevent the development of chronic inflammatory conditions, which can compromise the immune system over time.

Detoxification Support: The detoxifying effect of iodine extends to the removal of biological and environmental toxins that can impair immune function. By promoting the excretion of harmful substances, iodine reduces the burden on the immune system, allowing it to focus on defending against pathogens rather than dealing with toxins.

Enhancing Antioxidant Defense: Iodine contributes to the body's antioxidant defense system by supporting the activity of selenium-based enzymes, which protect cells from oxidative stress. Oxidative stress can weaken the immune system and make the body more susceptible to infections and chronic diseases. By mitigating oxidative damage, iodine indirectly strengthens immune resilience.

To harness these immune-boosting benefits of iodine, consider the following practical steps:

1. **Evaluate Your Iodine Intake:** Assess your diet to ensure it includes iodine-rich foods such as seaweed, fish, dairy products, and eggs. If your diet is lacking, consider iodine supplements, but consult with a healthcare provider to determine the appropriate dosage.

2. **Monitor Thyroid Function:** Since iodine's effects on the immune system are largely mediated through thyroid hormones, keeping an eye on thyroid health is crucial. Regular check-ups can help detect any imbalances early on.

3. **Incorporate Supporting Nutrients:** To maximize iodine's benefits, include other nutrients that support thyroid and immune health in your diet. Selenium, zinc, and vitamin D are particularly important and work synergistically with iodine.

4. **Stay Hydrated:** Adequate hydration supports all bodily functions, including detoxification processes facilitated by iodine. Aim for at least 8 glasses of water a day to help transport iodine throughout the body and assist in toxin removal.

5. **Exercise Regularly:** Physical activity boosts overall immune function and helps regulate thyroid hormones. Incorporating regular exercise into your routine can amplify the immune-supportive effects of iodine.

By understanding and applying these principles, individuals can effectively utilize iodine to fortify their immune system, enhancing their body's ability to resist infections and mitigate chronic health issues.

Reclaiming Your Energy

Fatigue and low energy levels can significantly impact your quality of life, making even simple daily tasks feel daunting. The key to **reclaiming your energy** lies in addressing the root causes of chronic tiredness, with a particular focus on optimizing thyroid health through adequate iodine intake. This essential mineral plays a crucial role in the synthesis of thyroid hormones, which regulate metabolism, energy production, and overall vitality.

Understanding Metabolic Rate and Thyroid Function: The thyroid gland orchestrates the body's metabolic rate through the production of hormones like thyroxine (T4) and triiodothyronine (T3). Insufficient iodine levels can lead to decreased production of these hormones, slowing down metabolic processes and resulting in persistent fatigue. Ensuring an adequate intake of iodine can support the thyroid in maintaining a healthy metabolic rate, thereby enhancing energy levels.

Strategies for Enhancing Energy with Iodine:

1. **Evaluate Dietary Sources:** Incorporate iodine-rich foods into your diet, such as seaweed, dairy products, eggs, and fish. These natural sources can help boost your iodine intake and support thyroid function.

2. **Consider Supplementation:** If dietary adjustments are not sufficient to correct iodine deficiency, consider iodine supplements. It's essential to consult with a healthcare provider to determine the appropriate dosage, as excessive iodine can also disrupt thyroid function.

3. **Monitor Iodine Levels:** Regular testing of iodine levels can provide valuable insights into your body's needs and help you adjust your intake accordingly. This proactive approach ensures that your thyroid receives the necessary support to function optimally.

4. **Support with Selenium:** Selenium is another crucial nutrient for thyroid health, working in tandem with iodine to facilitate the production and conversion of thyroid hormones. Including selenium-rich foods like Brazil nuts, sunflower seeds, and fish in your diet can amplify the benefits of iodine.

5. **Hydration and Detoxification:** Adequate hydration is vital for overall health and can aid in the detoxification processes supported by iodine. Drinking plenty of water helps to flush out toxins that may contribute to fatigue.

6. **Exercise Regularly:** Physical activity stimulates thyroid hormone production and increases sensitivity to these hormones, effectively boosting metabolism and energy levels. Find an exercise routine that you enjoy and can maintain consistently.

7. **Manage Stress:** Chronic stress can lead to adrenal fatigue, which often co-occurs with thyroid issues, exacerbating energy depletion. Techniques such as meditation, yoga, and deep breathing can help manage stress levels and support overall endocrine health.

8. **Sleep Quality:** Ensuring sufficient, high-quality sleep is essential for the body to repair and regenerate. Poor sleep can disrupt thyroid function and further deplete energy levels. Establish a regular sleep schedule and create a restful environment to promote deep, restorative sleep.

By addressing iodine intake and supporting thyroid health, you can take significant steps toward reclaiming your energy and improving your metabolism. Remember, the journey to enhanced vitality is personal and may require adjustments along the way. Listening to your body and working closely with healthcare professionals can help you find the right balance and strategies to achieve optimal energy levels and overall well-being.

Brain Function and Mental Clarity

The impact of iodine on cognitive functions and mental clarity cannot be overstated. This essential mineral plays a critical role in the development and maintenance of brain health, influencing cognitive abilities and protecting against cognitive decline. The brain utilizes iodine for sustaining neurotransmitter synthesis, which is crucial for memory, learning, and reasoning processes. A deficiency in this vital nutrient can lead to a foggy brain, memory lapses, and a decreased ability to process information, underscoring the importance of ensuring adequate intake for optimal mental performance.

Iodine's Role in Neurological Health is multifaceted. It contributes to the myelination of the central nervous system, which is essential for the rapid transmission of signals between neurons. Myelin acts as an insulating layer around nerves, and without sufficient iodine, this process can be compromised, leading to slower cognitive functions and impaired neural communication. Moreover, iodine's antioxidant properties help protect brain cells from oxidative stress, a contributing factor to neurodegenerative diseases such as Alzheimer's and Parkinson's.

To **Support Brain Function and Mental Clarity** through iodine, consider the following strategies:

1. **Incorporate Iodine-Rich Foods**: Seafood, such as fish, seaweed, and shellfish, are excellent sources of iodine. Dairy products and eggs also contribute to dietary iodine intake. Including these foods in your diet can help maintain adequate iodine levels, supporting brain health.

2. **Consider Supplementation if Necessary**: For individuals unable to meet their iodine needs through diet alone, supplements can be an effective way to ensure adequate intake. It's crucial to consult with a healthcare provider before starting any

supplementation, as they can recommend the appropriate dosage based on individual needs and avoid the risk of over-supplementation.

3. **Monitor Iodine Intake**: Both deficiency and excess iodine can have adverse effects on cognitive function. Regular monitoring of iodine levels can help maintain a balance that supports brain health without tipping into potentially harmful territory.

4. **Pair Iodine with Other Nutrients**: Selenium, zinc, and omega-3 fatty acids are other nutrients that play supportive roles in brain health. Selenium, for example, works synergistically with iodine to support antioxidant defense systems in the brain. Ensuring a balanced intake of these nutrients can enhance the cognitive benefits of iodine.

5. **Stay Hydrated**: Adequate hydration is essential for overall brain function. Water facilitates the transport of iodine throughout the body, including to the brain, and helps in the elimination of toxins that can impair cognitive function.

6. **Regular Exercise**: Physical activity increases blood flow to the brain, supporting the delivery of iodine and other nutrients essential for cognitive health. Exercise also stimulates the production of neurotrophic factors, which are involved in the growth and maintenance of neuronal connections.

By understanding the critical role iodine plays in brain function and mental clarity, individuals can take proactive steps to support their cognitive health. Ensuring adequate iodine intake through diet or supplementation, in conjunction with a healthy lifestyle, can provide a solid foundation for maintaining mental sharpness and protecting against cognitive decline.

PART 4: Special Applications of Iodine

Chapter 9: Iodine for Women's Health

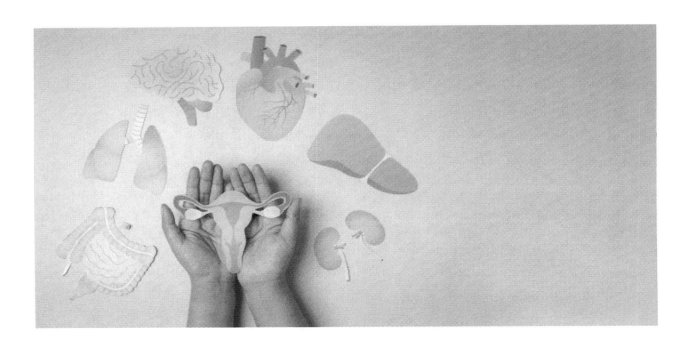

Breast Health and Hormonal Balance

For women, maintaining breast health and achieving hormonal balance are crucial aspects of overall well-being, and the role of iodine in these areas cannot be overstated. Iodine, a vital nutrient, has been shown to support breast tissue health and regulate hormonal functions, providing a natural approach to managing conditions such as fibrocystic breast disease and hormonal imbalances during menopause.

Fibrocystic Breast Disease: Many women experience fibrocystic breast changes, characterized by lumpiness and discomfort in the breast tissue. These changes are often linked to hormonal fluctuations. Iodine supplementation can be beneficial as it helps modulate the sensitivity of breast tissue to estrogen, reducing cyst formation and discomfort. A daily intake of iodine, in consultation with a healthcare provider, can support the normalization of breast tissue and alleviate the symptoms associated with fibrocystic breast disease.

Menopause and Hormonal Balance: The transition to menopause can be challenging, with symptoms like hot flashes, mood swings, and weight gain, largely due to hormonal imbalances. Iodine plays a pivotal role in the production of thyroid hormones, which regulate metabolism, mood, and body temperature. Ensuring adequate iodine intake supports thyroid function, which in turn can help manage menopausal symptoms more effectively. It's important to monitor iodine levels and adjust intake accordingly to support hormonal balance during this transition.

Dietary Sources of Iodine: Incorporating iodine-rich foods into the diet is a natural way to support breast health and hormonal balance. Sea vegetables, such as kelp, nori, and wakame, are excellent sources of iodine. Fish, dairy products, and eggs also contribute to iodine intake. For those who may not get enough iodine from their diet, supplements can be considered, but it's essential to choose the right type and dosage in consultation with a healthcare professional.

Supplemental Iodine: When dietary intake is insufficient, iodine supplements can be a valuable addition to support women's health. The form of iodine, dosage, and duration of supplementation should be personalized based on individual health needs and under the guidance of a healthcare provider. Monitoring iodine levels through appropriate testing is recommended to ensure optimal benefits while avoiding excessive intake.

Supporting Nutrients: For iodine to be most effective in supporting breast health and hormonal balance, it should be accompanied by adequate intake of other nutrients. Selenium, for example, is crucial for the optimal functioning of the thyroid gland and can enhance the benefits of iodine. Magnesium and vitamin D also play supportive roles in hormonal health and should be part of a comprehensive approach to wellness.

In conclusion, iodine is a key nutrient for women's health, particularly in supporting breast health and achieving hormonal balance. By understanding the importance of iodine and incorporating it appropriately into one's health regimen, women can navigate the challenges of fibrocystic breast disease and menopause more effectively. As always, consultation with a healthcare provider is essential to tailor iodine intake to individual health needs and ensure the best outcomes.

Iodine During Pregnancy

During pregnancy, the demand for iodine significantly increases, making it crucial for expectant mothers to ensure they are receiving an adequate supply. This essential nutrient plays a vital role in the development of the fetal brain and nervous system. The American Thyroid Association recommends that pregnant women consume at least 150 micrograms of iodine daily, a target that can be challenging to meet through diet alone, especially in areas where iodine deficiency is common.

Iodine's Impact on Fetal Development: Adequate iodine intake during pregnancy supports the development of the fetal nervous system and is critical for the synthesis of thyroid hormones, which are essential for brain development. A deficiency in this crucial period can lead to cretinism, a severe form of physical and intellectual disability.

Sources of Iodine for Pregnant Women: To meet the increased demands, pregnant women should focus on incorporating iodine-rich foods into their diet. Seafood, such as fish and shellfish, along with dairy products and eggs, are excellent sources. Additionally, iodized salt is a primary source of dietary iodine for many people. However, reliance solely on table salt for iodine can be problematic due to varying consumption levels and potential dietary restrictions.

Supplementation During Pregnancy: Given the critical nature of iodine for fetal development, many healthcare providers recommend iodine supplements as a part of prenatal care, especially for those who may not get enough from their diet. It is important to choose supplements specifically designed for pregnancy to ensure the correct dosage and to avoid exceeding the upper limit, which can lead to thyroid dysfunction.

Monitoring Iodine Intake: While ensuring adequate iodine intake is crucial, it is equally important to avoid excessive consumption, which can be harmful. Pregnant women should work closely with their healthcare provider to monitor their iodine levels, particularly if they are using supplements, to ensure they are within a safe range.

Adjusting Diet and Lifestyle: Beyond supplements, expectant mothers can enhance their iodine intake through mindful dietary choices. Incorporating a variety of iodine-rich foods and being cautious with the consumption of goitrogens, substances found in certain foods like soy and cruciferous vegetables that can interfere with iodine uptake, are practical steps that can be taken.

Educational Outreach: Awareness and education about the importance of iodine during pregnancy are key. Healthcare providers should inform pregnant women about the critical role of iodine in fetal development and provide guidance on achieving adequate intake through both diet and supplementation.

Pregnant women should always consult with their healthcare provider before starting any new supplement, including iodine, to ensure it is necessary and to determine the appropriate dosage. Tailoring iodine intake to individual needs, considering dietary sources, and possibly supplementing under medical supervision, are steps that can significantly impact the health and development of the baby.

Chapter 10: Iodine for Men's Health

Prostate Health and Iodine's Role

The prostate gland, a critical component of the male reproductive system, can be profoundly influenced by dietary and nutritional factors, including the intake of iodine. This trace element, essential for thyroid function, also plays a pivotal role in maintaining prostate health. Research suggests that adequate levels of this nutrient may contribute to a reduced risk of prostate issues, which become increasingly common as men age. Understanding the connection between iodine and prostate health, alongside implementing strategies for maintaining optimal iodine levels, can offer men a proactive approach to supporting their prostate health.

Iodine's Impact on Prostate Health

Iodine's anti-inflammatory and antioxidant properties make it beneficial for prostate health. It helps in modulating estrogen metabolism in the body, which is significant because estrogen dominance is a factor that can contribute to prostate enlargement and discomfort. By ensuring a balanced hormonal environment, iodine aids in maintaining prostate health and function.

Strategies for Optimizing Iodine Intake

1. **Dietary Sources**: Incorporating iodine-rich foods into one's diet is the first step towards ensuring adequate intake. Seafood, such as fish, shellfish, and seaweed, are excellent sources of iodine. Dairy products and eggs also contribute to dietary iodine, albeit to a lesser extent. For individuals with dietary restrictions or allergies, exploring plant-based sources like cranberries and strawberries, or iodine-fortified foods, can be beneficial.

2. **Supplementation**: For those unable to meet their iodine needs through diet alone, supplements can be a viable option. Iodine supplements come in various forms, including potassium iodide and nascent iodine. It's crucial to consult with a healthcare provider

before starting any supplementation to determine the appropriate type and dosage, as individual needs can vary based on overall health, diet, and lifestyle.

3. **Monitoring Iodine Levels**: Regular monitoring of iodine levels can help in adjusting intake to meet the body's needs. Simple urine tests are available and can provide insight into whether one's iodine intake is adequate, insufficient, or excessive. This is particularly important when using supplements, as both deficiency and excess iodine can impact health.

4. **Lifestyle Considerations**: Factors such as smoking and excessive alcohol consumption can negatively affect prostate health. Adopting a healthy lifestyle that includes regular physical activity, stress management, and avoiding toxins can complement iodine's beneficial effects on the prostate.

5. **Synergistic Nutrients**: Selenium, zinc, and vitamin D are other nutrients that play supportive roles in prostate health. Selenium, in particular, works synergistically with iodine, enhancing its thyroid and hormonal benefits. Ensuring adequate intake of these nutrients, either through diet or supplements, can amplify iodine's positive impact on prostate health.

Tailoring Iodine Intake

Personal health history, dietary habits, and lifestyle factors all influence the amount of iodine one needs. Men with a history of thyroid issues or autoimmune diseases should approach iodine supplementation with caution and under medical supervision. Similarly, those with a family history of prostate health issues may benefit from a tailored iodine intake plan that considers their specific risk factors and nutritional needs.

Implementing these strategies requires a commitment to regular health check-ups and an openness to adjusting one's diet and lifestyle as needed. With the right approach, iodine can be a valuable ally in maintaining prostate health and overall well-being.

Testosterone and Vitality

Testosterone, a crucial hormone in men, plays a vital role in maintaining muscle mass, bone density, and libido. Its production is significantly influenced by various factors, including diet, lifestyle, and nutrient intake, with iodine being a key element in this complex process. The thyroid gland, which requires iodine to produce hormones properly, indirectly affects testosterone levels. An imbalance in thyroid function can lead to alterations in hormone levels, including testosterone, thereby impacting a man's vitality and overall well-being.

Optimizing Testosterone Levels Through Iodine

1. **Ensure Adequate Iodine Intake**: Men should aim to consume the recommended daily allowance of iodine, which is 150 micrograms for adults. This can be achieved through a diet rich in iodine-containing foods such as seaweed, dairy products, eggs, and fish. For those who struggle to meet their iodine needs through diet alone, supplementation might be considered, under the guidance of a healthcare professional.

2. **Monitor Thyroid Function**: Regular check-ups with a healthcare provider can help monitor thyroid health and its impact on testosterone levels. If iodine deficiency is detected, addressing it can help normalize thyroid function, which in turn may stabilize testosterone levels.

3. **Lifestyle Modifications**: Engaging in regular exercise, particularly resistance and high-intensity interval training, can boost testosterone levels. Additionally, maintaining a healthy weight, managing stress through mindfulness practices, and ensuring adequate sleep are critical for optimal hormone production.

4. **Limit Exposure to Endocrine Disruptors**: Chemicals found in plastics, personal care products, and pesticides can interfere with hormone balance. Limiting exposure to these substances by choosing natural products and organic foods when possible can support hormonal health.

5. **Support with Other Nutrients**: Selenium, zinc, and vitamin D also play supportive roles in both thyroid and testosterone health. Ensuring sufficient intake of these nutrients, alongside iodine, can synergize to optimize hormone balance and vitality.

6. **Avoid Excessive Iodine**: While adequate iodine is crucial, excessive intake can have adverse effects on thyroid health and by extension, testosterone levels. It's important to find a balance and avoid surpassing the upper limit of 1,100 micrograms per day for adults.

The Role of Iodine in Energy and Vitality

Beyond its impact on testosterone, iodine plays a direct role in energy metabolism. The thyroid hormones, for which iodine is essential, regulate metabolic rate, energy production, and oxygen consumption in cells. An optimal level of iodine supports efficient metabolic function, contributing to a feeling of vitality and reducing fatigue.

Incorporating Iodine for Enhanced Well-being

- **Dietary Focus**: Emphasize iodine-rich foods in your diet. Sea vegetables like kelp and nori, fish such as cod and tuna, and even a moderate use of iodized salt can help meet iodine requirements.

- **Supplementation**: If dietary sources are insufficient, consider iodine supplements after consulting with a healthcare provider to determine the right form and dosage for your individual needs.

- **Holistic Approach**: Combine iodine optimization with other health-promoting practices. A balanced diet, regular physical activity, stress management, and adequate sleep form the cornerstone of hormonal health and vitality.

By addressing iodine intake and ensuring thyroid health, men can support their testosterone levels and overall vitality. This holistic approach not only enhances physical well-being but also contributes to mental and emotional health, underscoring the importance of iodine in men's health.

Chapter 11: Iodine for Youth Health

Brain Development Support

The significance of iodine in the development of a child's brain cannot be overstated. This essential nutrient plays a pivotal role in the synthesis of thyroid hormones, which are crucial for brain development and cognitive function. During the early years of life, the brain is in a rapid phase of growth and development. Ensuring adequate iodine intake during this period is vital for supporting neurological growth and preventing developmental disorders.

Iodine's Role in Neurological Development

Iodine contributes to the development of the nervous system in several critical ways. First, it is instrumental in the formation of myelin, the protective sheath around nerves that facilitates the quick and efficient transmission of electrical signals. Second, thyroid hormones, which depend on iodine for their production, regulate gene expression in the brain, influencing neural differentiation and maturation. Lastly, these hormones play a role in the migration of neurons during brain development, a process essential for the proper organization of the brain.

Identifying Adequate Iodine Intake

For children, the recommended daily intake of iodine varies by age:
- Ages 1-3: 90 micrograms (mcg) per day
- Ages 4-8: 90 mcg per day
- Ages 9-13: 120 mcg per day

Parents and caregivers can ensure children meet their iodine needs through a balanced diet that includes iodine-rich foods. Seafood, dairy products, and iodized salt are primary sources. For those with dietary restrictions or allergies, consulting with a healthcare provider about supplementation may be necessary.

Supporting Brain Health with Diet

Incorporating a variety of iodine-rich foods into a child's diet supports optimal brain development. Fish such as cod and tuna, dairy products like milk and yogurt, and even small amounts of iodized salt added to food can contribute to meeting daily requirements. Additionally, seaweed snacks, often rich in iodine, can be a child-friendly option.

Monitoring and Adjusting Iodine Intake

While iodine deficiency can lead to cognitive impairments and developmental delays, excessive intake can also be harmful, potentially leading to thyroid dysfunction. Regular check-ups with a pediatrician can help monitor a child's iodine status, especially if supplements are being used. Urinary iodine concentration tests offer a non-invasive method to assess iodine levels, guiding dietary adjustments as needed.

Educational Strategies for Parents

Understanding the importance of iodine in a child's diet is the first step toward ensuring adequate intake. Parents and caregivers can benefit from educational resources provided by healthcare professionals, including dietitians and pediatricians, on how to incorporate iodine-rich foods into meals and recognize signs of deficiency. Cooking classes, nutrition workshops, and school-based health programs can also offer practical strategies for supporting children's health through diet.

Collaboration with Healthcare Providers

For children with existing health conditions or those who are not meeting developmental milestones, collaboration with healthcare providers is essential. A tailored approach to iodine supplementation, guided by medical advice, can address specific needs without risking overexposure. Healthcare providers can also offer resources for tracking dietary intake and symptoms, ensuring a comprehensive approach to supporting brain development.

Ensuring that children receive adequate iodine through their diet or supplements is a critical component of supporting their overall development and cognitive function. By focusing on balanced nutrition, monitoring iodine status, and collaborating with healthcare professionals, parents and caregivers can contribute significantly to the neurological health and well-being of their children.

ADHD and Autism: Iodine's Neurobehavioral Benefits

In the realm of neurobehavioral conditions such as ADHD (Attention Deficit Hyperactivity Disorder) and autism spectrum disorders, emerging research suggests a potential link between iodine intake and symptom management. These conditions, characterized by challenges in social skills, repetitive behaviors, speech, and nonverbal communication, as well as issues with focus and hyperactivity, have been at the forefront of parental and medical concern for decades. While the exact causes of ADHD and autism are complex and multifaceted, involving genetic, environmental, and neurological factors, nutrition, including iodine intake, plays a crucial role in brain development and function.

Iodine is an essential micronutrient vital for the synthesis of thyroid hormones, which regulate metabolism and are critical for brain development and function. During the early stages of life, adequate iodine levels are paramount for neurodevelopment. Deficiencies in this nutrient can lead to a range of cognitive impairments and increased risk of learning disabilities. For children and adolescents with ADHD or autism, ensuring optimal iodine intake could support neurological health and mitigate some behavioral symptoms associated with these conditions.

1. **Thyroid Function and Neurodevelopment**: Thyroid hormones, fueled by iodine, are instrumental in brain development and cognitive function. Abnormalities in thyroid function can exacerbate or mimic symptoms of neurobehavioral disorders.

2. **Dietary Sources of Iodine**: Incorporating iodine-rich foods into the diet is a foundational step in managing ADHD and autism symptoms. Seafood, dairy products, eggs, and iodized salt are excellent sources. Seaweed, such as kelp, is particularly high in iodine and can be easily added to the diet in small amounts.

3. **Supplementation Considerations**: For individuals unable to meet their iodine needs through diet alone, supplementation may be necessary. However, it's crucial to consult with a healthcare provider to determine the appropriate dosage, as excessive iodine intake can lead to adverse effects, including worsening thyroid problems.

4. **Monitoring Iodine Intake**: Regular monitoring of iodine levels, especially in children and adolescents with ADHD or autism, can help ensure they are receiving an adequate but not excessive amount. This can be done through urinary iodine concentration tests, which provide a snapshot of iodine intake.

5. **Supporting Nutrients**: Alongside iodine, other nutrients such as selenium, zinc, and omega-3 fatty acids play supportive roles in brain health and function. A balanced diet rich in these nutrients can complement iodine intake and support overall neurological health.

6. **Individualized Approach**: Given the variability in dietary needs and the potential for underlying health conditions, an individualized approach to iodine supplementation and dietary modification is essential. Collaborating with healthcare professionals specializing in nutrition and neurodevelopmental disorders can provide tailored guidance.

7. **Research and Advocacy**: Continued research into the role of iodine and other dietary factors in ADHD and autism is crucial. Advocacy for nutritional education and support for affected families can empower them to make informed decisions about their health and well-being.

In summary, while iodine alone is not a cure for ADHD or autism, its role in supporting thyroid function and neurological health makes it an important consideration in the comprehensive management of these conditions. By ensuring adequate iodine intake through diet or supplementation, in consultation with healthcare providers, parents and caregivers can support the neurodevelopmental health of their children, potentially reducing the severity of symptoms associated with ADHD and autism.

Safe Doses for Kids

Ensuring the well-being of children involves careful consideration of their nutritional needs, including the intake of essential micronutrients such as iodine. This trace element plays a pivotal role in the development and functioning of the thyroid gland, which in turn supports growth, brain development, and metabolism in children and adolescents. However, determining the **safe doses** for this age group requires an understanding of their unique physiological needs and potential sensitivities.

For infants up to 6 months, the recommended dietary allowance (RDA) is set at 110 micrograms (mcg) per day. This amount typically comes from breast milk or formula, assuming the mother or the formula is adequately iodized. From 7 to 12 months, the RDA slightly increases to 130 mcg per day. It's important for parents and caregivers to ensure that infants receive an adequate supply of iodine, as deficiencies at this critical stage can lead to irreversible cognitive impairments.

As children grow, their need for iodine increases. Children aged 1-8 years should aim for an intake of 90 mcg per day. This can be achieved through a balanced diet that includes iodine-rich foods such as fish, dairy products, and iodized salt. For those aged 9-13 years, the RDA goes up to 120 mcg per day. Adolescents, from 14 years and older, require as much iodine as adults, which is 150 mcg per day. It's during these years that attention to dietary sources becomes crucial, especially for those following diets that may limit iodine-rich foods, such as vegan or dairy-free diets.

Supplementation should be approached with caution and always under the guidance of a healthcare professional. While iodine is vital, excessive intake can lead to conditions such as hyperthyroidism or contribute to the development of autoimmune thyroid diseases. For children and adolescents who require supplementation, it's generally advised not to exceed the tolerable upper intake levels (UL) established by health authorities. For children 1-3 years, the UL is set at 200 mcg per day; for those 4-8 years, it's 300 mcg; for ages 9-13 years, the UL is 600 mcg; and for adolescents 14-18 years, it's 900 mcg per day.

Monitoring the iodine status of children and adolescents involves observing for signs of deficiency or excess. Symptoms of deficiency can include poor growth, learning difficulties, and lethargy, while signs of excess might manifest as swelling in the neck (due to goiter) or unexpected weight loss. Regular check-ups with a healthcare provider can help in assessing iodine status through clinical evaluation and, if necessary, urine tests for iodine concentration.

Incorporating iodine into the diet of children and adolescents can be done through thoughtful meal planning. Including seafood once or twice a week, using iodized salt in cooking, and choosing dairy products are practical ways to ensure adequate intake. For those with dietary restrictions, consulting with a dietitian can help in identifying alternative sources of iodine, such as eggs, bread made with iodized salt, or iodine-fortified foods.

Parents and caregivers play a crucial role in monitoring and adjusting the iodine intake of their children to support optimal growth and development. Collaborating with healthcare professionals to tailor iodine intake, whether through diet or supplementation, ensures that the specific needs of each child or adolescent are met, safeguarding their health and well-being.

Chapter 12: Preventing and Treating Cancer with Iodine

Iodine and Breast Cancer Prevention

Breast cancer, a prevalent concern among women worldwide, has been the subject of extensive research to uncover preventive measures and supportive therapies. Among the various elements analyzed, iodine has emerged as a significant factor due to its potential role in both the prevention of breast cancer and as a supportive element in treatment protocols. The thyroid gland, which utilizes iodine to produce hormones, plays a crucial role in regulating the body's metabolism, including the rate at which cells grow and divide. Given the thyroid's influence on cell proliferation, adequate iodine intake is hypothesized to be protective against the development of cancerous cells in breast tissue.

Iodine's Mechanism in Breast Health: At the cellular level, iodine contributes to apoptosis, the process of programmed cell death, which is essential for eliminating damaged or cancerous cells. This mechanism suggests that iodine may help in reducing the risk of breast cells becoming cancerous. Furthermore, iodine is known for its anti-inflammatory and antioxidant properties, offering additional protective effects against cancer development.

Research Findings: Studies have indicated a correlation between low iodine intake and an increased risk of breast cancer. Women in regions with iodine-deficient soils and consequently lower dietary iodine intake appear to have higher rates of breast cancer. Conversely, populations consuming diets rich in iodine, such as those with a high intake of seaweed and other sea vegetables, show lower incidences of the disease.

Iodine Supplementation and Breast Health: For individuals looking to incorporate iodine into their wellness regimen for breast health, it's crucial to approach supplementation with care. The body's iodine needs are relatively small, and while deficiency can pose health risks, excessive intake can lead to thyroid dysfunction. Consulting with a healthcare provider to determine the appropriate dosage based on individual health status and dietary iodine intake is essential.

Dietary Sources of Iodine: Incorporating iodine-rich foods into the diet is a practical approach to ensuring adequate intake. Seafood, dairy products, and iodized salt are common sources. Seaweed, such as kelp, nori, and wakame, stands out for its high iodine content and can be easily added to a variety of dishes.

Supporting Nutrients: Selenium, zinc, and vitamin D are among the nutrients that enhance iodine's effectiveness and support overall breast health. Selenium, in particular, works synergistically with iodine in thyroid hormone synthesis and metabolism. Ensuring a balanced intake of these nutrients can optimize the protective effects of iodine against breast cancer.

Considerations for Women with Existing Thyroid Conditions: Women with thyroid disorders, such as hypothyroidism or autoimmune thyroiditis, should exercise caution when adjusting their iodine intake. Since iodine metabolism is closely linked to thyroid function, changes in iodine levels can impact thyroid disease. Close monitoring by a healthcare professional is advisable for women with these conditions who are considering iodine supplementation for breast health.

Monitoring Iodine Status: Regular assessment of iodine levels can help in maintaining an optimal balance. Urinary iodine concentration tests offer a means to monitor iodine status and adjust dietary intake or supplementation as needed. This proactive approach ensures that iodine contributes to breast health without adversely affecting thyroid function.

Incorporating iodine into a comprehensive strategy for breast cancer prevention and support involves understanding its multifaceted role in the body's metabolic processes and its potential impact on breast tissue health. Balancing iodine intake through diet or supplementation, in conjunction with a healthcare provider's guidance, offers a proactive measure for supporting breast health and reducing cancer risk.

Skin Cancer Applications

The therapeutic potential of iodine in the context of skin cancer, both through topical and systemic applications, presents a compelling avenue for adjunctive treatment strategies. The antiseptic properties of iodine, long recognized for their effectiveness in disinfecting wounds, also extend to a capability to induce apoptosis in cancerous cells without harming the surrounding healthy tissue. This dual action makes iodine a unique candidate for skin cancer management.

Topical Application: The direct application of iodine on skin lesions has been observed to exert a cytotoxic effect on cancerous cells. For basal cell and squamous cell carcinomas, the most common types of non-melanoma skin cancers, topical iodine can be applied in a diluted form to the affected area. The concentration and frequency of application should be carefully monitored to avoid skin irritation, with a typical starting point being a 2% iodine solution applied once daily, gradually increasing based on tolerance and response.

Systemic Application: Beyond topical use, iodine's systemic effects on skin health and cancer prevention are linked to its role in apoptosis and the regulation of the cell cycle. Oral intake of iodine supplements can contribute to a systemic approach to skin cancer prevention, particularly in individuals with low dietary iodine intake. The recommended daily allowance (RDA) for adults is 150 micrograms, but in cases of deficiency or for therapeutic purposes, higher doses may be considered under medical supervision. It's crucial to maintain a balance, as excessive iodine can disrupt thyroid function and lead to adverse health outcomes.

Supporting Skin Health with Iodine-Rich Diet: Incorporating iodine-rich foods into one's diet is another strategy to support skin health and potentially reduce the risk of skin cancer. Seafood, dairy products, and iodized salt are excellent sources of iodine. For individuals with dietary restrictions, seaweed snacks or supplements can provide an alternative source of this essential micronutrient.

Adjunctive Nutrients for Enhanced Efficacy: To optimize the benefits of iodine for skin health, it's beneficial to include other nutrients that support skin integrity and immune function. Selenium, vitamin C, and zinc, for example, can enhance iodine's efficacy and provide additional antioxidant and immune-boosting effects. A balanced intake of these nutrients, alongside iodine, contributes to a comprehensive approach to skin cancer prevention and treatment.

Monitoring and Adjustments: It's important for individuals using iodine for skin cancer treatment or prevention to regularly monitor their skin's response to treatment and adjust their strategy accordingly. This includes observing for any signs of irritation or adverse reactions to topical applications and adjusting the concentration or frequency of use as needed. For systemic applications, monitoring thyroid function and overall health is essential to ensure that iodine supplementation remains within safe limits.

Collaboration with Healthcare Providers: Whether considering topical or systemic applications of iodine for skin cancer, collaboration with healthcare providers is paramount. This ensures that the use of iodine is tailored to the individual's specific health profile, skin cancer type, and overall treatment plan. Healthcare providers can offer guidance on the appropriate form, dosage, and application method of iodine, as well as monitor for efficacy and safety throughout the treatment process.

Incorporating iodine into the management and prevention of skin cancer involves a nuanced understanding of its mechanisms of action, potential benefits, and the importance of balance and monitoring. With careful application and oversight, iodine presents a promising adjunctive strategy in the fight against skin cancer, offering hope for both prevention and improved outcomes in treatment.

Part 5: Resources and Tools

Chapter 13: FAQs About Iodine

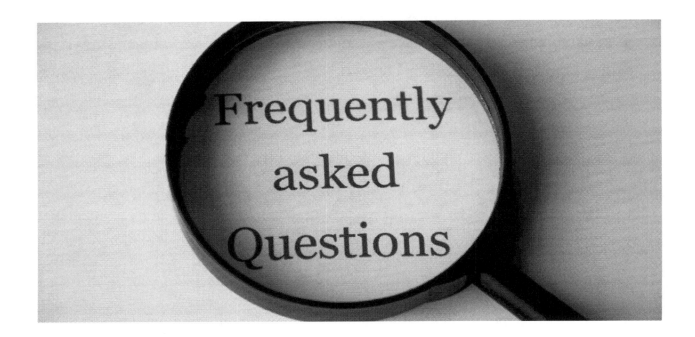

Common Concerns

When considering the addition of iodine to your regimen for thyroid health, detoxification, immunity enhancement, or energy improvement, several common concerns arise. These include questions about safety, appropriate dosages, and practical applications. Addressing these concerns with factual, evidence-based information is crucial to making informed decisions about your health.

Safety of Iodine Supplementation: The safety of iodine supplementation largely depends on individual health status and existing iodine levels. For most individuals, iodine is a critical nutrient that supports numerous bodily functions, especially thyroid health. However, it's important to approach supplementation with caution, as both deficiency and excess can lead to health issues. The key is to maintain a balance. Individuals with thyroid disorders, such as Hashimoto's thyroiditis or Graves' disease, should consult healthcare professionals before starting any form of supplementation, as iodine can impact these conditions in complex ways.

Determining the Right Dosage: The appropriate dosage of iodine can vary significantly among individuals, depending on factors like age, weight, dietary intake, and health status. The Recommended Dietary Allowance (RDA) for adults is 150 micrograms (mcg) per day, but therapeutic doses, especially for detoxification purposes, may be higher. It's imperative to start with a lower dose and gradually increase it if necessary, under the guidance of a healthcare provider. Monitoring your body's response to supplementation and adjusting the dosage accordingly is essential to avoid potential side effects such as thyroid dysfunction or iodine toxicity.

Practical Applications of Iodine: Incorporating iodine into your health regimen doesn't solely rely on supplements. A diet rich in iodine-containing foods, such as seaweed, fish, dairy products, and eggs, can significantly contribute to your daily intake. For those focusing on detoxification, understanding the role of iodine in eliminating toxins like heavy metals, fluoride, and bromide is crucial. Combining iodine supplementation with other supportive strategies, such as adequate hydration, a balanced diet rich in antioxidants, and possibly the use of salt loading to facilitate bromide excretion, can enhance detoxification processes.

Addressing Iodine Deficiency: Identifying iodine deficiency involves recognizing symptoms such as fatigue, weight gain, cold intolerance, and swelling of the thyroid gland (goiter). If deficiency is suspected, a healthcare provider can confirm it through tests such as urinary iodine concentration. Addressing deficiency requires a careful increase in iodine intake, either through diet or supplementation, with regular monitoring to avoid overshooting to iodine excess.

Avoiding Overuse and Side Effects: While iodine is essential, overuse can lead to adverse effects, including thyroid gland inflammation, hyperthyroidism, or hypothyroidism. Signs of excessive iodine intake include palpitations, anxiety, sleep disturbances, and changes in thyroid function tests. If you experience any of these symptoms, it's important to reevaluate your iodine dosage with a healthcare professional and make necessary adjustments.

Incorporating iodine into your health regimen for thyroid support, detoxification, immunity boosting, or energy enhancement requires a balanced approach. Understanding the safety considerations, determining the right dosage for your individual needs, and applying iodine effectively through both diet and supplementation are key steps in leveraging the benefits of this essential nutrient. Always consult with a healthcare provider to tailor the approach to your specific health profile and goals, ensuring that iodine serves as a beneficial component of your overall wellness strategy.

Chapter 14: Advanced Protocols and Testing

Why Personalization Matters

Personalizing your iodine detoxification protocol is crucial due to the unique nature of each individual's health status, toxin exposure, and personal health goals. Understanding that there is no one-size-fits-all approach to detoxification, especially when it comes to using iodine, is the first step in crafting a plan that addresses your specific needs effectively.

Exposure to Toxins: Your daily exposure to toxins plays a significant role in determining the right approach to iodine detoxification. Factors such as living in a high-pollution area, occupational hazards, or the frequent consumption of processed foods can increase your body's toxin load. A higher exposure level might necessitate a more aggressive detox plan compared to someone with minimal exposure.

Health Conditions: Pre-existing health conditions, particularly those related to thyroid health, necessitate a tailored approach to iodine supplementation. For instance, individuals with Hashimoto's thyroiditis may require a different protocol than those with hypothyroidism without autoimmune involvement. Consulting with a healthcare provider to understand the nuances of your condition is essential.

Personal Health Goals: Your objectives, whether it's improving energy levels, enhancing thyroid function, or supporting overall detoxification, influence the choice and dosage of iodine. Goals focused on long-term health maintenance might favor a gradual approach, while acute health issues could benefit from a more structured protocol.

Iodine Sensitivity: Sensitivity to iodine varies among individuals, with some experiencing adverse reactions at lower doses. Starting with a low dose and gradually increasing it allows you to monitor your body's response and adjust accordingly.

Nutritional Support: Accompanying nutrients, such as selenium, magnesium, and vitamin C, can enhance the effectiveness of iodine and mitigate potential side effects. Personalizing your supplement regimen to include these supportive nutrients is key to a successful detox.

Lifestyle Factors: Daily habits, including diet, hydration, and exercise, can influence the effectiveness of your iodine detox plan. Incorporating iodine-rich foods, ensuring adequate water intake, and engaging in regular physical activity can support the detoxification process.

In summary, personalizing your iodine detoxification approach is essential for maximizing benefits while minimizing risks. By considering your unique exposure to toxins, health conditions, personal health goals, iodine sensitivity, nutritional needs, and lifestyle factors, you can develop a comprehensive and effective detox plan. Regular monitoring and adjustments, guided by feedback from your body and healthcare professionals, will ensure that your detoxification journey is both safe and beneficial.

Types of Detox Programs

Light Detox for Beginners

Embarking on a light detoxification regimen with iodine is an excellent starting point for individuals who have minimal exposure to toxins and are new to the concept of using this essential element for health enhancement. This approach involves a conservative intake of 1-3 milligrams of iodine per day, equivalent to approximately 1-2 drops of Lugol's 2% solution. This modest dosage is designed to gently initiate the body's detoxification processes without overwhelming it, making it an ideal choice for beginners.

Hydration plays a pivotal role in this detoxification phase. Adequate water intake is crucial as it facilitates the flushing out of toxins and supports the kidneys in their filtration functions. It is recommended to drink at least eight 8-ounce glasses of water daily, though individual needs may vary based on factors such as body weight and activity level. Incorporating water-rich foods into one's diet, such as cucumbers, tomatoes, and watermelons, can also contribute to overall hydration and enhance the detoxification process.

A light diet complements this detox phase, focusing on foods that are easy on the digestive system and rich in nutrients that support detoxification and overall health. Emphasis should be placed on organic fruits and vegetables, lean proteins, and whole grains. These foods provide essential vitamins, minerals, and antioxidants that aid in the detoxification process. Cruciferous vegetables like broccoli, Brussels sprouts, and kale are particularly beneficial due to their high content of compounds that support liver health and detoxification.

Seafood, a natural source of iodine, can be included in the diet to provide an additional boost of this critical nutrient. However, it is important to select low-mercury options such as wild-caught salmon, sardines, and trout to avoid adding to the body's toxic burden. Seaweed and other sea vegetables are also excellent sources of iodine and can be easily incorporated into meals in the form of salads, soups, or snacks.

During this light detox phase, it is essential to listen to your body and be attentive to how it responds to the increased iodine intake. Some individuals may experience mild detoxification symptoms, such as slight fatigue or headaches, which typically indicate that the body is adjusting and beginning to eliminate stored toxins. These symptoms are generally transient and can be alleviated by ensuring adequate hydration and rest.

It is also beneficial to engage in gentle physical activities, such as walking or yoga, which support the body's natural detoxification processes through increased circulation and perspiration. However, it is crucial to avoid overexertion during this phase to prevent undue stress on the body.

In summary, a light detoxification protocol with iodine is a prudent and effective way to begin cleansing the body of accumulated toxins. By adhering to a regimen of low-dose iodine supplementation, proper hydration, and a nutrient-rich diet, individuals can gently support their body's natural detoxification pathways. This approach lays a solid foundation for achieving improved thyroid health, enhanced immunity, and greater overall vitality.

Moderate Detox with Lugol's and Nutritional Support

For individuals ready to elevate their detoxification efforts beyond the foundational stage, a moderate detox regimen offers a more intensive approach to purging toxins from the body, leveraging a higher dosage of iodine, the implementation of the Salt Loading Protocol, and the strategic inclusion of supportive nutrients such as selenium and vitamin C. This phase is designed for those who have acclimated to the initial iodine intake and are seeking to deepen the detoxification process, targeting a more thorough removal of accumulated toxins.

Increasing the iodine dosage to 5-10 milligrams daily, equivalent to approximately 4-8 drops of Lugol's 2% solution, intensifies the body's ability to flush out toxins. This heightened dosage serves to more aggressively mobilize stored toxins from tissues, facilitating their excretion. It is crucial, however, to proceed with this increased dosage cautiously, monitoring the body's response closely to avoid potential detoxification symptoms that may arise from the more rapid release of toxins.

The Salt Loading Protocol emerges as a pivotal component in this phase, aimed at enhancing the elimination of bromide and fluoride, two common halides that compete with iodine for absorption and utilization in the body. By ingesting a solution of high-quality, unrefined salt dissolved in water, followed by additional plain water to encourage hydration, this method accelerates the excretion of displaced halides through the urine. The protocol typically involves consuming 1/4 to 1/2 teaspoon of salt dissolved in 8 ounces of water, followed by at least 12 ounces of additional water, repeated as necessary to facilitate toxin removal. It is a critical step in mitigating potential detoxification reactions and ensuring the effective elimination of unwanted substances from the body.

Nutritional support plays a significant role in this enhanced detoxification strategy. Selenium, an essential trace element, works synergistically with iodine, supporting efficient thyroid function and providing antioxidant protection against oxidative stress induced by toxin mobilization. A daily intake of 200 micrograms of selenium is recommended to bolster the body's defense mechanisms during this detox phase. Vitamin C, known for its potent antioxidant properties, further aids in neutralizing free radicals and supports the immune system in handling the increased toxin load. A daily dosage of 1,000 to 3,000 milligrams of vitamin C, divided into multiple doses throughout the day to maximize absorption and utilization, can significantly enhance the body's resilience against the oxidative stress of detoxification.

Adhering to this moderate detox regimen requires a mindful approach, with attention to the body's signals and readiness to adjust dosages as needed. It is advisable to introduce the increased iodine dosage gradually, allowing the body to adapt to its enhanced detoxifying role. Similarly, the Salt Loading Protocol should be tailored to individual tolerance levels, with adjustments made based on the body's response and the effectiveness of toxin elimination as evidenced by symptom relief and overall well-being.

Incorporating these strategies into a comprehensive detox plan, while ensuring adequate hydration, balanced nutrition, and regular physical activity, sets the stage for a successful moderate detoxification experience. This phase represents a critical step in the journey toward optimal health, offering a pathway to more profound healing and revitalization through the strategic use of iodine, targeted nutritional support, and effective toxin elimination practices.

Intensive Detox for Deep Toxin Removal

For individuals who have navigated through the foundational and moderate stages of iodine detoxification, an intensive detox regimen represents a significant escalation in the effort to purge deep-seated toxins from the body. This phase is tailored for those who, after careful assessment and under medical supervision, are prepared to tackle a more profound level of toxin removal. The intensive detox protocol necessitates the administration of iodine in dosages ranging from 15 to 50 milligrams daily. Such quantities are designed to mobilize and excrete toxins that have been deeply embedded in tissues and organs over time.

The necessity for medical supervision cannot be overstated in this context. The elevated dosages used in this phase carry the potential for more pronounced detoxification symptoms and require a healthcare professional's guidance to navigate safely. Medical oversight ensures that the detox process is both effective and does not compromise the individual's health. Physicians or healthcare providers specializing in detoxification and holistic health are best suited to oversee this intensive protocol. They can offer invaluable insights into adjusting dosages, managing symptoms, and interpreting the body's responses to the treatment.

At this stage, the body's reaction to the increased iodine intake must be meticulously monitored. Symptoms such as heightened fatigue, skin reactions, or changes in thyroid function tests may indicate the body's response to the mobilization of toxins. These signs require careful evaluation to distinguish between normal detoxification responses and potential adverse effects. Adjustments to the protocol may be necessary based on these observations, emphasizing the personalized nature of an intensive detox plan.

Supporting the body with additional nutrients becomes even more critical in this phase. The role of selenium continues to be paramount, given its protective effects against oxidative stress and its contribution to maintaining thyroid health. Magnesium and vitamin C, along with a well-rounded multivitamin, can further assist in managing the increased oxidative load and supporting the body's detoxification pathways. Ensuring an adequate intake of antioxidants through diet or supplementation can help mitigate some of the detoxification symptoms and promote overall well-being.

Hydration remains a cornerstone of the detoxification process, with increased water intake essential to facilitate the excretion of toxins. The Salt Loading Protocol, previously introduced, may be adjusted in frequency and quantity to enhance its effectiveness in this more intensive phase. The aim is to optimize the elimination of bromide and fluoride, which are displaced by iodine from their cellular binding sites.

Dietary considerations during this phase should focus on maximizing the intake of organic, nutrient-dense foods that support detoxification. Foods rich in fiber, such as fruits, vegetables, and whole grains, can aid in the elimination of toxins through the digestive tract. Incorporating foods high in natural iodine, like seaweed and other sea vegetables, can complement the iodine supplementation and provide a broad spectrum of minerals beneficial for detoxification.

Engaging in light to moderate physical activity can support the detoxification process by promoting circulation and encouraging the elimination of toxins through sweat. However, the intensity and duration of exercise should be carefully modulated to avoid overburdening the body during this intensive detox phase.

In this advanced stage of detoxification, the emphasis on a holistic approach becomes even more pronounced. The integration of mind-body practices such as meditation, yoga, or tai chi can provide stress relief and enhance the body's resilience against the challenges of intensive detoxification. These practices not only support physical detoxification but also promote mental and emotional well-being, facilitating a more comprehensive healing experience.

The intensive detox phase is a commitment to deep healing and requires a structured, well-monitored approach to achieve its objectives safely. With the right support, careful planning, and adherence to medical guidance, individuals can navigate this challenging yet rewarding phase towards achieving optimal health and vitality.

Managing Detox Symptoms

Common Symptoms

When individuals embark on an iodine detoxification regimen, they may experience a range of symptoms indicative of the body's natural response to the elimination of stored toxins. Among the most commonly reported symptoms are headaches, fatigue, and joint pain. These manifestations can serve as signals from the body that it is adjusting to the changes induced by increased iodine intake and the mobilization of toxins from tissues.

Headaches during a detox phase can often be attributed to the release of toxins from the body's stores, which then circulate in the bloodstream before being excreted. This process can temporarily increase the toxic load on the body, potentially leading to discomfort and pain. Adequate hydration is crucial in this context, as it facilitates the flushing out of toxins through the kidneys and can help alleviate headache symptoms. Drinking water, along with herbal teas known for their detoxifying properties, such as dandelion or milk thistle tea, can be particularly beneficial.

Fatigue is another symptom commonly experienced during the detoxification process. As the body expends energy to mobilize and eliminate toxins, individuals may feel unusually tired or lethargic. Supporting the body with nutrients that enhance energy production can be helpful. For instance, incorporating foods rich in B-vitamins, such as whole grains, nuts, and seeds, can support energy metabolism. Additionally, ensuring adequate sleep and rest during this period allows the body to regenerate and recover, thereby mitigating feelings of fatigue.

Joint pain is a symptom that some individuals may encounter as the body detoxifies. This discomfort can result from the inflammatory response to toxins being released from storage sites, including the joints. To address this, incorporating anti-inflammatory foods into the diet can be advantageous. Omega-3 fatty acids, found in fatty fish, flaxseeds, and walnuts, have been shown to possess anti-inflammatory properties that may help alleviate joint pain. Furthermore, gentle physical activities such as stretching, yoga, or swimming can help maintain joint mobility and reduce discomfort.

It's important for individuals undergoing an iodine detox to listen to their bodies and adjust their detoxification protocols as needed. If symptoms become severe or persist, it may be necessary to reduce the iodine dosage temporarily or consult with a healthcare provider for further guidance. The use of supportive therapies, such as massage or acupuncture, may also provide relief from detox symptoms and enhance the body's natural healing processes.

In managing these common symptoms, the goal is to support the body's detoxification efforts while minimizing discomfort. This holistic approach not only addresses the physical aspects of detoxification but also considers the individual's overall well-being. Through careful management of symptoms and supportive care, individuals can navigate the detoxification process more comfortably, paving the way for improved health and vitality.

Relief Strategies

When embarking on an iodine detoxification protocol, it's not uncommon to experience a range of detox symptoms, including headaches, fatigue, and joint pains. These manifestations, while temporary, can be uncomfortable and may deter some from continuing with their detox journey. However, there are effective relief strategies that can help mitigate these symptoms, ensuring a more comfortable and sustainable detox process.

One of the most effective methods for alleviating detox symptoms is the use of Epsom salt baths. Epsom salt, a mineral compound comprised of magnesium and sulfate, is renowned for its ability to soothe muscle aches, reduce inflammation, and promote relaxation. When dissolved in warm bath water, the magnesium and sulfate are absorbed through the skin, directly targeting areas of discomfort. For optimal results, it's recommended to indulge in an Epsom salt bath for at least 20 minutes. This not only aids in relieving pain but also supports the body's detoxification pathways by facilitating the excretion of toxins through the skin.

In addition to Epsom salt baths, adopting an anti-inflammatory diet plays a crucial role in managing detox symptoms. This dietary approach focuses on consuming foods that are known to reduce inflammation, thereby alleviating discomfort and enhancing overall well-being. Key components of an anti-inflammatory diet include a variety of colorful fruits and vegetables, rich in antioxidants and phytonutrients, lean protein sources, healthy fats, and whole grains. Foods particularly beneficial for their anti-inflammatory properties include berries, leafy greens, nuts, seeds, and fatty fish such as salmon and mackerel. Conversely, it's advisable to limit the intake of processed foods, sugars, and trans fats, as these can exacerbate inflammation and hinder the detoxification process.

Hydration is another critical element in managing detox symptoms effectively. Drinking ample amounts of water throughout the day facilitates the elimination of toxins through urine and sweat. Furthermore, incorporating herbal teas, such as ginger or peppermint tea, can offer additional relief from symptoms like nausea and digestive discomfort.

For those experiencing significant detox symptoms, it may be beneficial to adjust the dosage of iodine temporarily. Lowering the dose can help reduce the intensity of symptoms, making the detox process more manageable. It's important to listen to your body's signals and adjust accordingly, always prioritizing comfort and safety.

Lastly, engaging in gentle physical activities such as walking, yoga, or stretching can further support the detoxification process. These activities promote circulation, enhance lymphatic drainage, and contribute to overall physical and mental well-being.

By implementing these relief strategies, individuals undergoing an iodine detox can effectively manage symptoms, ensuring a smoother and more comfortable detoxification experience. It's essential to approach detox with patience and self-care, recognizing that the process is a positive step towards restoring health and vitality.

When to Stop

Recognizing the signs that indicate it's time to halt or adjust your iodine supplementation is crucial for maintaining optimal health and preventing adverse effects. While iodine plays a vital role in supporting thyroid function, detoxification, and overall well-being, there is a fine line between beneficial and potentially harmful dosages. This section delves into the critical indicators that suggest your body may not be tolerating the current level of iodine intake well, necessitating a reduction in dosage or a complete cessation of supplementation.

Swelling in the Neck: One of the first signs of excessive iodine intake can be swelling in the neck, where the thyroid gland is located. This swelling, known as a goiter, occurs as the thyroid attempts to process the surplus iodine. If you notice any unusual enlargement in your neck, it's imperative to consult with a healthcare professional and reassess your iodine dosage.

Thyroid Function Disruption: Excessive iodine can lead to either hyperthyroidism or hypothyroidism, conditions characterized by the overactive or underactive function of the thyroid gland, respectively. Symptoms of hyperthyroidism include unexpected weight loss, rapid heartbeat, increased appetite, and anxiety. Conversely, signs of hypothyroidism encompass fatigue, weight gain, cold intolerance, and depression. Any sudden or unexplained changes in weight, mood, or energy levels should prompt a reevaluation of iodine intake.

Skin Rash or Acne: A sudden onset of acne or a skin rash might also signal that the body is not responding favorably to the amount of iodine being consumed. These skin manifestations can be a direct reaction to iodine detoxification processes, indicating that the body is attempting to eliminate excess iodine through the skin.

Digestive Disturbances: Experiencing gastrointestinal issues such as nausea, stomach pain, or diarrhea shortly after increasing iodine supplementation could indicate that your body is struggling to process the excess iodine. Digestive discomfort associated with iodine supplementation should not be overlooked.

Metallic Taste or Dry Mouth: A metallic taste in the mouth or an unusually dry mouth can be subtle signs of excessive iodine intake. These symptoms may appear relatively minor but are worth noting as indicators that your iodine levels may need adjustment.

In the presence of these symptoms, it's advisable to immediately reduce or halt iodine supplementation and seek guidance from a healthcare provider. A professional can assess your symptoms, conduct necessary thyroid function tests, and recommend an appropriate course of action based on your individual health status.

Adjusting iodine intake is not a one-size-fits-all process; it requires careful monitoring and personalization. For some, a temporary reduction in iodine may suffice, while others may need to discontinue use altogether to allow the body to rebalance. It's essential to approach iodine supplementation with a mindset of flexibility and attentiveness to your body's cues, ensuring that this powerful nutrient remains a beneficial part of your health regimen rather than a source of discomfort or harm.

Practical Detox Tools

Checklist for Choosing the Right Protocol

Embarking on an iodine detoxification regimen requires careful consideration of various factors to ensure that the chosen protocol aligns with individual health status, exposure to toxins, and personal wellness goals. The following checklist is designed to guide individuals through the process of selecting the most appropriate detoxification strategy, taking into account their unique circumstances and needs.

1. **Assess Your Current Health Status**: Before initiating any detox plan, it's crucial to evaluate your overall health. Consider any existing conditions, particularly those related to thyroid health, such as hypothyroidism or autoimmune thyroid disorders. Understanding your health baseline will help in tailoring the detox approach to avoid exacerbating any pre-existing conditions.

2. **Determine Your Exposure Level to Toxins**: The extent of your exposure to environmental toxins, including heavy metals, fluoride, and bromide, plays a significant role in choosing the right detox protocol. Those with minimal exposure may benefit from a lighter detox regimen, while individuals with significant toxin exposure might require a more intensive approach.

3. **Identify Personal Health Goals**: Clarify what you aim to achieve through iodine detoxification. Whether it's enhancing thyroid function, boosting immunity, or improving energy levels, your goals will influence the intensity and duration of the detox protocol.

4. **Consider Iodine Sensitivity**: Recognize any signs of iodine sensitivity or adverse reactions to iodine-containing foods or supplements in the past. This awareness is vital for adjusting the dosage and form of iodine to minimize potential side effects.

5. **Evaluate Nutritional Support**: The success of an iodine detox plan is significantly enhanced by concurrent nutritional support. Ensure the inclusion of essential nutrients such as selenium, magnesium, and vitamin C in your diet or supplementation regimen, as these elements support thyroid health and aid in the detoxification process.

6. **Lifestyle Factors**: Your daily habits, including diet, hydration levels, and physical activity, can impact the effectiveness of the detox protocol. A diet rich in organic fruits and vegetables, adequate water intake, and regular, gentle exercise can support the body's natural detox pathways.

7. **Select the Type of Iodine Supplement**: Based on the above considerations, choose the most suitable form of iodine supplement. Options include Lugol's solution, nascent iodine, or potassium iodide, each with different absorption rates and effects on the body.

8. **Determine the Starting Dosage**: Starting with a low dose and gradually increasing it allows your body to adjust to the iodine and minimizes detox symptoms. The initial dosage should be decided based on your sensitivity, health goals, and level of toxin exposure.

9. **Plan for Symptom Management**: Be prepared to manage detox symptoms such as headaches, fatigue, or skin reactions. Strategies may include Epsom salt baths, an anti-inflammatory diet, and adjustments to the iodine dosage based on your body's response.

10. **Monitor Your Progress**: Keep a detailed journal of your symptoms, dietary intake, and any changes in your health status. Regular monitoring will help in adjusting the detox protocol as needed and tracking improvements over time.

11. **Consult Healthcare Professionals**: Seek guidance from healthcare providers knowledgeable about iodine use and detoxification. Their expertise can be invaluable in customizing the detox plan to your specific needs and ensuring safety throughout the process.

By meticulously following this checklist, individuals can select an iodine detoxification protocol that is both safe and effective, tailored to their health status and wellness objectives. This personalized approach facilitates optimal results, enhancing thyroid function, detoxification, and overall well-being without compromising safety.

Tracking Your Progress

Monitoring your progress during an iodine detoxification process is an essential component of managing and optimizing your health outcomes. This involves detailed tracking of both the physical and emotional changes you experience, which can provide invaluable insights into how your body is responding to the detox. By keeping a comprehensive record, you can identify patterns, understand the efficacy of the detox protocol, and make informed adjustments as necessary to enhance your overall well-being.

To effectively track your progress, start by establishing a baseline of your symptoms and general health status before beginning the detox. This baseline should include a detailed list of any thyroid-related symptoms, such as fatigue, weight changes, mood fluctuations, and other relevant health markers. Additionally, note your current dietary habits, hydration levels, physical activity routines, and any supplements or medications you are taking. This initial snapshot of your health will serve as a crucial point of reference throughout the detox process.

As you embark on your iodine detox, create a daily log to record various aspects of your health and well-being. This log should include:

1. **Symptom Severity and Frequency**: Note any existing symptoms and any new symptoms that emerge. Rate the severity of these symptoms on a scale that makes sense to you, such as 1 to 10, and track how frequently they occur. This can help you discern whether your symptoms are improving, worsening, or remaining stable over time.

2. **Dietary Intake**: Keep a detailed record of your food and fluid intake, emphasizing iodine-rich foods, hydration levels, and any changes you make to your diet in response to the detox. This information can help you correlate dietary patterns with changes in your symptoms or overall health.

3. **Supplement Dosage**: Document the type and amount of iodine supplementation you are using, along with any other supportive nutrients or supplements. Adjustments to your

supplementation regimen should be noted, as these can significantly impact your detox experience and outcomes.

4. **Physical and Emotional Well-being**: Beyond physical symptoms, it's important to monitor your emotional and mental health. Changes in mood, energy levels, sleep patterns, and stress levels can all provide insights into how the detox is affecting your overall well-being.

5. **Lifestyle Factors**: Record any modifications to your lifestyle, such as increases in physical activity, implementation of stress-reduction techniques, or adjustments to your sleep routine. These factors can play a critical role in supporting your body's detoxification efforts and can influence the effectiveness of the iodine detox.

6. **Detox Symptoms and Relief Strategies**: If you experience detox symptoms, document these alongside any relief strategies you employ, such as Epsom salt baths, dietary adjustments, or changes in supplementation. This information can be invaluable for managing discomfort and for identifying what strategies are most effective for you.

7. **Healthcare Consultations**: Keep a record of any consultations with healthcare professionals, including their recommendations and any adjustments to your detox protocol. This ensures that you have a comprehensive overview of the medical guidance you receive and how it aligns with your detox journey.

By maintaining a detailed and organized log of your iodine detoxification process, you empower yourself with the knowledge and insights needed to tailor the detox to your unique health needs. This proactive approach allows for timely adjustments to your protocol, ensuring that you are supporting your body in the most effective and safe manner possible. Remember, the goal of tracking your progress is not only to observe improvements but also to recognize when modifications are necessary to optimize your health outcomes. This diligent monitoring is a testament to your commitment to achieving optimal thyroid health, detoxification, and overall vitality through the strategic use of iodine.

Chapter 15: Iodine-Rich Diet Recipes

Simple Iodine-Rich Recipes

1. **Seaweed Salad with Sesame Dressing**
   - Soak 1 cup of mixed seaweed in water for 20 minutes. Drain and squeeze out excess water.
   - Whisk together 2 tablespoons soy sauce, 1 tablespoon sesame oil, 1 tablespoon rice vinegar, and 1 teaspoon honey.
   - Toss the seaweed with the dressing and sprinkle with sesame seeds before serving.

2. **Baked Cod with Iodine-Rich Crust**
   - Mix 1/2 cup crushed seaweed snacks, 1/4 cup breadcrumbs, and 1 teaspoon lemon zest.
   - Brush 4 cod fillets with olive oil and press the seaweed mixture onto one side.
   - Bake at 400°F for 12-15 minutes or until the fish flakes easily.

3. **Iodine-Boost Smoothie**
   - Blend 1 banana, 1/2 cup Greek yogurt, 1/4 cup cranberries, 1 tablespoon spirulina, and 1 cup almond milk until smooth.

4. **Kelp Noodle Stir Fry**
   - Rinse and prepare 1 package of kelp noodles as per package instructions.
   - Stir-fry your choice of vegetables (bell peppers, broccoli, carrots) in sesame oil and add noodles with 2 tablespoons of soy sauce and 1 tablespoon of oyster sauce.
   - Cook until the vegetables are tender and the noodles are heated through.

5. **Iodine-Rich Egg Salad**
   - Hard boil 6 eggs, then peel and chop.
   - Mix with 1/4 cup mayonnaise, 1 tablespoon mustard, 1/2 teaspoon dulse granules, salt, and pepper.
   - Serve on whole-grain bread with lettuce.

6. Seaweed Chips

- Toss 2 cups of kale and 1 cup of torn nori sheets with 1 tablespoon of olive oil and sea salt.
- Bake at 300°F for 10-15 minutes until crispy.

7. Miso Soup with Wakame

- Dissolve 2 tablespoons of miso paste in 4 cups of simmering water.
- Add 1/2 cup soaked wakame, tofu cubes, and sliced green onions.
- Simmer for 5 minutes before serving.

8. Roasted Brussels Sprouts with Iodized Salt

- Toss 2 cups of halved Brussels sprouts with olive oil and sprinkle with iodized salt.
- Roast at 400°F for 20-25 minutes, stirring halfway through.

9. Shrimp and Avocado Salad

- Mix 1 pound cooked shrimp, 1 diced avocado, 1/2 cup chopped tomatoes, and 1/4 cup diced red onion.
- Dress with lime juice, olive oil, salt, and pepper.

10. Sardine Toast

- Mash 1 can of sardines with 1 tablespoon of mayonnaise and spread on toasted whole-grain bread.
- Top with sliced cucumber and a sprinkle of dulse flakes.

11. Quinoa Salad with Seaweed

- Cook 1 cup quinoa according to package instructions and let cool.
- Mix quinoa with 1/2 cup chopped seaweed, 1 diced bell pepper, 1/4 cup sliced green onions, and a dressing of lemon juice, olive oil, salt, and pepper.

12. Iodine-Rich Trail Mix

- Combine 1/2 cup dried cranberries, 1/2 cup roasted seaweed snacks, 1/2 cup nuts (almonds or cashews), and 1/4 cup pumpkin seeds.

13. Grilled Salmon with Teriyaki Glaze

- Marinate 4 salmon fillets in a mixture of 1/4 cup teriyaki sauce and 1 tablespoon minced ginger for 30 minutes.

- Grill on medium-high heat for 5-7 minutes per side.

14. Yogurt with Fresh Berries and Seaweed Granola

- Mix 1 cup plain Greek yogurt with 1/2 cup fresh berries.

- Top with 1/4 cup granola mixed with 1 tablespoon crushed seaweed snacks.

15. Sweet Potato and Seaweed Hash

- Sauté 1 diced sweet potato in olive oil until tender.

- Add 1/2 cup chopped onions and 1/4 cup rehydrated seaweed; cook until onions are translucent.

16. Iodine-Rich Vegetable Soup

- In a large pot, sauté 1 chopped onion, 2 diced carrots, and 2 diced celery stalks.

- Add 6 cups vegetable broth, 1 cup chopped kale, and 1/4 cup chopped seaweed.

- Simmer for 20 minutes.

17. Tuna Salad with Capers and Dulse

- Mix 1 can of tuna, 2 tablespoons mayonnaise, 1 tablespoon capers, and 1 teaspoon dulse flakes.

- Serve on whole-grain crackers.

18. Roasted Seaweed Stuffed Peppers

- Mix cooked quinoa, diced tomatoes, crumbled feta

Meal Plans for Thyroid and Detox

Thyroid-Boosting Breakfast Plan

Objective: To create a breakfast plan that supports thyroid function through iodine-rich foods, enhancing overall energy and well-being.

Step-by-step instructions:

1. **Begin with a Glass of Lemon Water**

   - Upon waking, drink a glass of warm water with the juice of half a lemon to kickstart your digestion and liver function.

2. **Seaweed Smoothie**

   - **Ingredients:** 1 cup of almond milk, 1 banana, 1 tablespoon of organic seaweed powder (like kelp or spirulina), a handful of spinach, and a tablespoon of chia seeds.

   - **Instructions:** Blend all ingredients until smooth. This smoothie is rich in iodine and antioxidants, supporting thyroid health and detoxification.

3. **Egg and Vegetable Scramble**

   - **Ingredients:** 2 organic eggs, ½ cup of diced vegetables (such as bell peppers, onions, and spinach), 1 teaspoon of coconut oil, and a sprinkle of kelp granules for an extra iodine boost.

   - **Instructions:** Sauté the vegetables in coconut oil until soft. Beat the eggs and pour them over the vegetables, cooking until the eggs are firm. Sprinkle with kelp granules before serving.

4. **Whole Grain Toast with Avocado**

   - **Ingredients:** 1 slice of whole-grain or gluten-free toast and ½ an avocado.

   - **Instructions:** Mash the avocado and spread it on the toast. Top with a pinch of sea salt and hemp seeds for added texture and nutrients.

5. Herbal Tea or Iodine Supplement

- **Option 1:** Enjoy a cup of herbal tea such as green tea or dandelion tea, which supports detoxification and hydration.

- **Option 2:** If advised by your healthcare provider, take an iodine supplement with your breakfast to ensure you're meeting your daily iodine needs.

6. Mindful Eating Practice

- Take at least 20 minutes to eat your breakfast without distractions. Focus on the flavors, textures, and sensations of eating, which aids in digestion and satisfaction.

7. Morning Sun Exposure

- After breakfast, spend 10-15 minutes outside in natural sunlight. Morning sun exposure helps regulate your circadian rhythm, supporting better energy levels throughout the day.

8. Hydration Reminder

- Finish your breakfast with another glass of water or herbal tea to stay hydrated. Proper hydration is crucial for thyroid health and detoxification processes.

This thyroid-boosting breakfast plan incorporates iodine-rich foods, hydration, and practices that support overall health and energy levels. Adjust portions and ingredients according to your personal preferences and nutritional needs.

Detoxifying Lunch Plan

Objective: To create a nutritious, iodine-rich lunch plan that supports detoxification and thyroid health, while also being delicious and satisfying.

Step-by-step instructions:

1. **Start with a Seaweed Salad:**

   - Soak 1 cup of mixed seaweed (like arame, wakame, or hijiki) in water for 10-15 minutes to rehydrate.

   - Drain and mix with sliced cucumber, diced avocado, and a handful of baby spinach.

   - Dress with a mixture of 2 tablespoons rice vinegar, 1 tablespoon sesame oil, a pinch of sea salt, and a sprinkle of sesame seeds.

2. **Prepare a Main Dish of Grilled Wild Salmon:**

   - Marinate a 6-ounce wild salmon fillet in a mixture of lemon juice, minced garlic, and dill for at least 30 minutes.

   - Grill the salmon on medium heat for 3-4 minutes per side, or until it flakes easily with a fork.

   - Serve with a side of steamed broccoli or asparagus, lightly seasoned with olive oil and lemon zest.

3. **Incorporate a High-Iodine Soup:**

   - In a pot, sauté 1 chopped onion, 2 minced garlic cloves, and 1 diced carrot in olive oil until soft.

   - Add 4 cups of vegetable broth, 1 cup of chopped tomatoes, and 1 cup of sliced mushrooms. Simmer for 20 minutes.

   - Stir in 1 cup of chopped kale and 1 tablespoon of kelp granules. Cook for an additional 5 minutes. Season with thyme, oregano, salt, and pepper to taste.

4. Choose a Detoxifying Beverage:

- Brew a cup of green tea, known for its antioxidant properties and a modest amount of natural iodine.

- Alternatively, prepare a fresh juice by blending 1 apple, 1 beet, a handful of spinach, and a small piece of ginger with water. This drink is rich in nutrients that support detoxification pathways.

5. End with a Light, Iodine-Rich Dessert:

- Mix 1/2 cup of plain Greek yogurt with 1 teaspoon of honey, a sprinkle of chopped nuts (like almonds or walnuts), and a few slices of fresh strawberry.

- Top with a small handful of dried cranberries or cherries for an added boost of antioxidants and a touch of natural sweetness.

Note: This lunch plan is designed to provide a balanced intake of iodine from natural food sources, along with other nutrients that support thyroid function and detoxification processes. Adjust portions and ingredients according to personal dietary needs and preferences.

Iodine-Rich Dinner Plan

Objective: To create a nutritious, iodine-rich dinner plan that supports thyroid health, aids in detoxification, and boosts energy levels. This meal plan is designed to be both delicious and beneficial for those looking to enhance their dietary intake of iodine through natural food sources.

Step-by-step instructions:

1. **Starter: Seaweed Salad**
   - Rinse a cup of mixed seaweed under cold water and soak for 5-10 minutes to rehydrate.
   - Drain and squeeze out excess water from the seaweed.
   - In a bowl, mix the seaweed with a dressing made from 2 tablespoons of sesame oil, 1 tablespoon of soy sauce, a dash of rice vinegar, and a sprinkle of sesame seeds.
   - Chill in the refrigerator for at least 30 minutes before serving to allow flavors to meld.

2. **Main Course: Baked Cod with Iodine-Rich Seasoning**
   - Preheat your oven to 375°F (190°C).
   - Take 4 cod fillets and place them in a baking dish.
   - In a small bowl, mix 1 teaspoon of sea salt, ½ teaspoon of garlic powder, ½ teaspoon of onion powder, and a pinch of ground black pepper.
   - Sprinkle the seasoning mix over the cod fillets.
   - Drizzle each fillet with a tablespoon of olive oil and bake for 12-15 minutes, or until the fish flakes easily with a fork.

3. **Side Dish: Roasted Brussels Sprouts with Kelp Flakes**
   - Preheat the oven to 400°F (200°C).
   - Trim and halve 2 cups of Brussels sprouts and place them on a baking sheet.
   - Toss the Brussels sprouts with 2 tablespoons of olive oil, salt, and pepper to taste.
   - Roast in the oven for 20-25 minutes, until crispy on the outside and tender on the inside.
   - Once out of the oven, sprinkle with 1 tablespoon of kelp flakes for an iodine boost.

4. Dessert: Greek Yogurt with Fresh Berries and Honey

   - Serve a cup of plain, full-fat Greek yogurt as a base.

   - Top the yogurt with a half-cup of mixed fresh berries (blueberries, strawberries, raspberries).

   - Drizzle with a tablespoon of raw honey for natural sweetness.

5. Beverage: Iodine-Infused Water

   - Fill a pitcher with filtered water.

   - Add slices of lemon and cucumber for flavor.

   - Incorporate a few drops of nascent iodine supplement into the water (as per the product's dosage recommendation).

   - Stir well and refrigerate to chill. Serve with dinner to enhance iodine intake.

Note: This dinner plan is designed to provide a balanced intake of iodine from natural food sources, complemented by the nascent iodine-infused water for an additional boost. Adjust portions and iodine supplement dosage according to individual dietary needs and preferences. Always consult with a healthcare provider before starting any new dietary supplement, especially if you have pre-existing health conditions or concerns.

Energy-Enhancing Snack Plan

Objective: To create a daily snack plan that boosts energy levels through the incorporation of iodine-rich foods, supporting thyroid health and enhancing detoxification processes.

Step-by-step instructions:

1. **Morning Snack**:

 - **Ingredients**: 1 medium banana, 1 tablespoon of organic seaweed flakes, and a handful of raw nuts (almonds or walnuts).

 - **Preparation**: Slice the banana and sprinkle with seaweed flakes. Serve with a side of raw nuts for a crunchy texture and an extra energy boost.

 - **Why It Works**: Bananas provide a quick source of natural sugar and energy, while seaweed flakes are rich in iodine, supporting thyroid function. Nuts add healthy fats and protein, stabilizing blood sugar levels until your next meal.

2. **Mid-Morning Snack**:

 - **Ingredients**: Greek yogurt (unsweetened), fresh berries (strawberries, blueberries, or raspberries), and a drizzle of honey.

 - **Preparation**: Mix a cup of Greek yogurt with a half-cup of fresh berries. Drizzle with a teaspoon of honey for a touch of sweetness.

 - **Why It Works**: Greek yogurt is high in protein, aiding in sustained energy levels. Berries provide antioxidants and a modest amount of sugar for an energy lift. The iodine in dairy supports thyroid health, while honey adds a quick energy spike.

3. **Afternoon Snack**:

 - **Ingredients**: 1 small apple, 2 tablespoons of almond butter, and a sprinkle of chia seeds.

 - **Preparation**: Slice the apple and spread almond butter over each slice. Sprinkle chia seeds on top for added texture and nutrients.

- **Why It Works**: Apples are high in fiber and provide a slow-releasing source of energy. Almond butter contributes healthy fats and protein, and chia seeds are rich in omega-3 fatty acids, enhancing overall energy production and endurance.

4. **Late Afternoon Snack**:
   - **Ingredients**: A small bowl of mixed seaweed salad (available at health food stores or Asian markets).
   - **Preparation**: If not pre-mixed, combine various types of seaweed like wakame, nori, and hijiki. Dress lightly with sesame oil and rice vinegar for flavor.
   - **Why It Works**: Seaweed is one of the best natural sources of iodine, crucial for thyroid health, which in turn regulates energy levels. The light dressing adds a flavorful twist without adding too many calories.

5. **Pre-Dinner Snack**:
   - **Ingredients**: Homemade trail mix with dried cranberries, pumpkin seeds, sunflower seeds, and unsweetened coconut flakes.
   - **Preparation**: Mix equal parts of each ingredient in a bowl. Store in an airtight container and serve a small cup as a snack.
   - **Why It Works**: This snack provides a balance of healthy fats, protein, and a small amount of natural sugars. Pumpkin seeds and sunflower seeds offer magnesium and zinc, supporting thyroid function and energy metabolism. Dried cranberries add a touch of sweetness and antioxidants, while coconut flakes provide a source of medium-chain triglycerides for a quick energy boost.

Note: Always ensure that the iodine-rich foods integrated into your snack plan are suitable for your individual health needs, especially if you have specific thyroid conditions. Consult with a healthcare provider if you are unsure about incorporating new foods into your diet.

Immune-Boosting Meal Plan

Objective: To create a 7-day immune-boosting meal plan that incorporates iodine-rich foods to support thyroid health, detoxification processes, and enhance overall energy levels. This plan is designed for health-conscious adults seeking practical and nutritious ways to integrate more iodine into their diets for improved immunity and vitality.

Step-by-step instructions:

1. **Day 1:**
   - **Breakfast:** Scrambled eggs with spinach and cheese. Use iodized salt for seasoning.
   - **Lunch:** Tuna salad with mixed greens, avocado, and a sprinkle of seaweed flakes.
   - **Dinner:** Grilled salmon with a side of roasted Brussels sprouts and quinoa.

2. **Day 2:**
   - **Breakfast:** Greek yogurt topped with strawberries and a small handful of nuts.
   - **Lunch:** Sardine and arugula sandwich on whole-grain bread with mustard and tomato slices.
   - **Dinner:** Baked chicken breast with steamed broccoli and sweet potato mash.

3. **Day 3:**
   - **Breakfast:** Oatmeal cooked in milk (or a milk alternative) with sliced banana and a dash of iodized salt.
   - **Lunch:** Quinoa salad with chickpeas, cucumber, feta cheese, and olives.
   - **Dinner:** Stir-fried shrimp with mixed vegetables (carrots, bell peppers, and snow peas) served over brown rice.

4. **Day 4:**
   - **Breakfast:** Smoothie made with kale, pineapple, banana, and flaxseed meal.
   - **Lunch:** Turkey and cranberry sauce wrap with spinach and cream cheese.
   - **Dinner:** Cod fillets baked with a crust of crushed almonds and herbs, served with asparagus and a side salad.

5. **Day 5:**

   - **Breakfast:** Two boiled eggs with whole-grain toast and a side of mixed berries.

   - **Lunch:** Lentil soup with carrots, celery, and onions, seasoned with iodized salt.

   - **Dinner:** Beef stir-fry with broccoli, bell peppers, and onions, served with a side of brown rice.

6. **Day 6:**

   - **Breakfast:** Chia pudding made with almond milk and topped with sliced mango and coconut flakes.

   - **Lunch:** Chicken Caesar salad with romaine lettuce, Parmesan cheese, and whole-grain croutons.

   - **Dinner:** Baked trout with lemon and dill, served with a quinoa and spinach salad.

7. **Day 7:**

   - **Breakfast:** Pancakes made with buckwheat flour, topped with a dollop of Greek yogurt and fresh blueberries.

   - **Lunch:** Avocado and egg salad sandwich on whole-grain bread.

   - **Dinner:** Roast lamb with rosemary and garlic, served with roasted root vegetables (carrots, parsnips, and beets).

Note: Throughout the week, ensure adequate hydration by drinking at least 8 glasses of water daily. Consider incorporating a daily multivitamin or specific supplements as recommended by a healthcare provider to support overall health and ensure adequate intake of all essential nutrients.

Metabolism-Revving Breakfast Plan

Objective: To create a breakfast plan that stimulates the metabolism, supports thyroid function, and enhances detoxification efforts through iodine-rich foods.

Step-by-step instructions:

1. **Begin with a Glass of Lemon Water:** Upon waking, drink a glass of warm water with the juice of half a lemon. This aids in hydration and kick-starts the liver detoxification process.

2. **Seaweed Smoothie:** Prepare a smoothie using 1 cup of almond milk, 1 banana, a handful of fresh spinach, 1 tablespoon of organic seaweed powder (such as kelp or spirulina), and a handful of blueberries. Seaweed is a natural source of iodine and antioxidants, while the banana and blueberries provide energy and fiber.

3. **Egg and Vegetable Scramble:** Cook 2 eggs with a mix of vegetables such as bell peppers, onions, and kale. Eggs are a good source of selenium, a nutrient that works synergistically with iodine to support thyroid health. The vegetables add essential vitamins and minerals, boosting the detoxification process.

4. **Whole-Grain Toast with Avocado:** Serve your scramble with a slice of whole-grain toast topped with mashed avocado. The whole grains provide sustained energy through complex carbohydrates, while the avocado offers healthy fats to support hormone balance and absorption of fat-soluble vitamins.

5. **Brazil Nuts for Selenium:** Finish your meal with 2 Brazil nuts. They are one of the richest sources of selenium, which is crucial for the efficient utilization of iodine in the body and overall thyroid health.

6. **Green Tea:** Sip on a cup of organic green tea. Green tea is rich in antioxidants, supports metabolism, and aids in detoxification. It's a gentle way to stimulate metabolism further without overwhelming the thyroid.

7. **Mindful Eating Practice:** While consuming your breakfast, focus on eating slowly and mindfully. This practice aids digestion and absorption of nutrients, ensuring your body gains the maximum benefit from this iodine-rich meal.

8. **Hydration Reminder:** Continue to drink water throughout the morning to stay hydrated. Proper hydration is essential for detoxification and to keep the metabolism functioning optimally.

By following this Metabolism-Revving Breakfast Plan, you're not only supporting your thyroid and boosting your metabolism but also taking significant steps towards enhancing your body's detoxification processes and overall energy levels.

Cleansing Lunch Plan

Objective:

Create a nutritious and iodine-rich lunch plan that supports thyroid health and detoxification, boosting immunity and energy levels.

Step-by-step instructions:

1. **Start with a Seaweed Salad:**

   - Soak 1 cup of mixed seaweed (such as wakame, arame, or kelp) in water for 5-10 minutes to rehydrate.

   - Drain and mix with a dressing made from 2 tablespoons of rice vinegar, 1 tablespoon of sesame oil, 1 teaspoon of honey, and a pinch of salt.

   - Add sliced cucumber, grated carrot, and a sprinkle of sesame seeds for extra crunch and nutrients.

2. **Prepare a Main Dish of Grilled Salmon:**

   - Marinate a 6-ounce salmon fillet in a mixture of lemon juice, minced garlic, and dill for at least 30 minutes.

   - Grill the salmon over medium heat for 3-4 minutes on each side or until it flakes easily with a fork.

   - Serve with a side of steamed broccoli or asparagus for a dose of fiber and antioxidants.

3. **Incorporate a Small Serving of Brown Rice:**

   - Cook 1/2 cup of brown rice according to package instructions.

   - Enhance the rice by stirring in a teaspoon of kelp granules and a tablespoon of chopped fresh parsley once cooked.

4. **Add a Detoxifying Beverage:**

   - Brew a cup of green tea, known for its antioxidant properties and a mild source of iodine.

   - Optionally, sweeten with a teaspoon of honey or enjoy plain to appreciate its natural flavors.

5. **Finish with a Fruit-Based Dessert:**

- Slice a medium-sized apple and serve with a tablespoon of almond butter for a satisfying end to your meal.

- The fiber in the apple and the healthy fats in the almond butter will aid digestion and keep you feeling full longer.

6. **Hydration Throughout the Meal:**

- Ensure you drink at least 8 ounces of filtered water during your meal to aid in digestion and detoxification.

- Consider adding a slice of lemon or cucumber to your water for added flavor and detoxifying benefits.

This lunch plan is designed to provide a balanced mix of iodine-rich foods, antioxidants, and nutrients that support thyroid function, detoxification processes, and overall health. Adjust portions according to your dietary needs and preferences.

Nutrient-Dense Dinner Plan

Objective: Create a nutrient-dense dinner plan that incorporates iodine-rich foods to support thyroid health and detoxification, boosting immunity and energy levels.

Step-by-step instructions:

1. **Select Your Main Protein Source:** Opt for wild-caught fish, such as cod or shrimp, known for their high iodine content. Aim for a 6-ounce serving per person. If you prefer a vegetarian option, consider baked tofu marinated in seaweed flakes.

2. **Choose Your Vegetables:** Focus on cruciferous vegetables like steamed broccoli or roasted Brussels sprouts, which support detoxification. Include a salad with dark leafy greens such as spinach or kale for an additional nutrient boost. Aim for at least 2 cups of vegetables per person.

3. **Incorporate Seaweed:** Add a side of seaweed salad or nori rolls as an appetizer. Seaweed is one of the richest sources of iodine and also provides fiber, which aids in detoxification.

4. **Select a Healthy Fat:** Cook your main dish and vegetables with coconut oil or dress your salad with a flaxseed oil-based vinaigrette. Both options will add healthy fats to your meal, enhancing the absorption of fat-soluble vitamins.

5. **Choose a Complex Carbohydrate:** Serve a side of quinoa or brown rice. Both are gluten-free grains that provide fiber and essential nutrients, complementing the iodine intake from other components of the meal. Aim for a ½ cup cooked serving per person.

6. **Prepare a Detoxifying Beverage:** Brew a cup of green tea or dandelion root tea for each person. These beverages support liver detoxification and provide antioxidants.

7. **End with an Iodine-Rich Dessert:** Offer a small serving of Greek yogurt topped with fresh strawberries and a sprinkle of chia seeds. This dessert provides additional iodine, probiotics, and antioxidants.

8. **Hydration:** Ensure that filtered water is available throughout the meal to aid in digestion and detoxification. Aim for at least one 8-ounce glass of water per person during the meal.

9. **Mindful Eating Practice:** Begin the meal with a moment of gratitude for the nourishment provided. Encourage slow, mindful eating to aid in digestion and absorption of nutrients.

10. **Post-Dinner Activity:** Conclude the evening with a gentle walk. Physical activity can aid digestion and promote a sense of well-being after a nutrient-dense meal.

Hydration-Focused Snack Plan

Objective: To create a daily snack plan focused on hydration and rich in iodine to support thyroid function and detoxification processes, enhancing overall energy and immunity.

Step-by-step instructions:

1. **Morning Snack:**

   - **Prepare a Smoothie:** Blend 1 cup of coconut water, 1 banana, 1/2 cup of frozen strawberries, and 1 tablespoon of cranberry juice (unsweetened). Coconut water is rich in electrolytes for hydration, while cranberries are a good source of iodine.

   - **Add a Boost:** Include 1 teaspoon of spirulina powder for an extra dose of iodine and antioxidants.

2. **Mid-Morning Snack:**

   - **Hydrating Fruit Bowl:** Combine 1/2 cup of cubed watermelon, 1/2 cup of sliced cucumbers, and a handful of fresh mint leaves. Both watermelon and cucumbers offer high water content and mint aids digestion.

   - **Iodine Sprinkle:** Top with a light drizzle of seaweed flakes to infuse an iodine boost.

3. **Afternoon Snack:**

   - **Crunchy Seaweed Snacks:** Opt for a pack of roasted seaweed snacks, readily available and rich in iodine. Pair with 1 cup of herbal tea or infused water (think cucumber or lemon slices in water) for hydration.

4. **Late Afternoon Snack:**

   - **Yogurt with Berries:** Mix 1 cup of Greek yogurt (plain, unsweetened) with 1/4 cup of mixed berries (blueberries, raspberries). Yogurt provides probiotics for gut health, and berries add hydration and antioxidants.

   - **Iodine and Fiber:** Sprinkle 1 tablespoon of chia seeds for fiber, which helps maintain hydration levels, and add a few drops of liquid iodine supplement as per your daily requirement.

5. Evening Snack:

  - **Vegetable Juice:** Make or buy a fresh vegetable juice consisting of carrots, beetroot, and a small piece of ginger. This combination is hydrating and rich in nutrients.

  - **Iodine Addition:** Stir in 1 teaspoon of powdered kelp or dulse for your iodine intake.

6. Throughout the Day:

  - **Stay Hydrated:** Aim to drink at least 8 glasses of water throughout the day. Consider infusing your water with slices of lemon, lime, or orange for added flavor and vitamin C, which can aid in the absorption of iodine.

  - **Mindful Snacking:** Listen to your body's hunger and fullness cues. These snacks are designed to be nutrient-dense and hydrating but adjust portions according to your individual needs and hunger levels.

Balanced Meal Plan for Thyroid Health

Objective: To create a balanced meal plan focused on supporting thyroid health through iodine-rich foods, while also incorporating other essential nutrients that aid in thyroid function and overall well-being.

Step-by-step instructions:

1. Breakfast: Thyroid-Boosting Smoothie

- Blend 1 cup of organic berries (strawberries, blackberries, and raspberries are great choices for their antioxidant properties), 1 banana for energy and sweetness, 1/2 cup of Greek yogurt for iodine and selenium, and a tablespoon of chia seeds for omega-3 fatty acids. Add a dash of seaweed powder for an extra iodine boost.

2. Mid-Morning Snack: Nutty Seaweed Snack

- Mix a handful of brazil nuts (rich in selenium) with dried seaweed snacks. This combination provides a crunchy, nutrient-dense snack that supports thyroid health.

3. Lunch: Quinoa Salad with Grilled Salmon

- Prepare a salad with cooked quinoa (a good source of zinc), mixed greens, sliced avocado (for healthy fats), and top with grilled salmon (rich in omega-3 fatty acids and iodine). Dress with a lemon vinaigrette for a refreshing taste.

4. Afternoon Snack: Cottage Cheese with Fresh Pineapple

- Combine 1/2 cup of cottage cheese (rich in iodine) with fresh pineapple chunks (for bromelain to aid digestion). This snack is not only satisfying but also supports thyroid function.

5. Dinner: Baked Chicken with Roasted Vegetables and Seaweed Gomasio

- Bake a chicken breast seasoned with herbs and serve with a side of roasted vegetables like broccoli, carrots, and sweet potatoes (all rich in fiber and essential vitamins). Sprinkle seaweed gomasio (a mix of sesame seeds, seaweed, and sea salt) over the dish for an iodine boost.

6. **Evening Snack: Iodine-Rich Fruit Compote**

- Gently cook diced apples and pears in a little water until soft. Add a sprinkle of cinnamon and a small handful of dried cranberries for added antioxidants. This light snack is soothing and beneficial for thyroid health.

7. **Hydration: Throughout the Day**

- Aim to drink at least 8 glasses of water throughout the day. Consider adding slices of lemon or cucumber for added flavor and detoxifying benefits. Staying well-hydrated is crucial for overall health and aids in the absorption of nutrients.

8. **Supplemental Support:**

- Consult with a healthcare provider about adding a daily multivitamin or specific supplements like selenium, zinc, and vitamin D to support thyroid health and ensure you're meeting your nutritional needs.

This balanced meal plan is designed to provide a comprehensive approach to supporting thyroid health through diet. Each meal and snack is crafted to include iodine-rich foods along with other nutrients essential for thyroid function and overall wellness. Remember, individual nutritional needs may vary, so it's important to adjust portions and ingredients as necessary to fit your personal health goals and dietary requirements.

Conclusion

Thriving with Iodine

Harnessing the power of iodine for your well-being is a transformative step toward achieving optimal health. This essential element plays a pivotal role in regulating thyroid function, which in turn influences your metabolic rate, energy levels, and immune system strength. By integrating iodine into your daily regimen, you're not just supporting thyroid health; you're laying the foundation for a more vibrant, energized life.

Understanding the significance of iodine in detoxification processes is crucial. It assists in the removal of harmful substances such as heavy metals and environmental toxins, which can accumulate in the body and lead to various health issues. Incorporating iodine-rich foods and supplements into your diet can enhance your body's natural detoxification pathways, promoting a cleaner, more efficient system.

Boosting your immunity is another remarkable benefit of maintaining adequate iodine levels. It supports the production and function of white blood cells, enhancing your body's ability to fight off infections and diseases. In a world where exposure to pathogens is inevitable, ensuring your immune system is robust is essential for maintaining health and preventing illness.

The impact of iodine on energy levels cannot be overstated. A well-functioning thyroid gland, supported by sufficient iodine intake, ensures that your body's energy production processes are running smoothly. This means you can enjoy sustained energy throughout the day, avoiding the common pitfalls of fatigue and lethargy that plague many.

To fully reap the benefits of iodine, it's important to identify the right type and dosage that aligns with your individual health needs. Whether it's through dietary sources like seaweed and dairy products or through supplementation, finding the balance that works for your body is key. Remember, consulting with a healthcare professional before making any significant changes to your supplement regimen is advisable to ensure safety and efficacy.

Supporting your iodine intake with other essential nutrients such as selenium, magnesium, and zinc can further enhance its benefits. These synergistic relationships not only maximize the positive effects on your thyroid and overall health but also help mitigate any potential risks associated with iodine supplementation.

As you continue to prioritize iodine in your health strategy, remember that consistency is key. Regular monitoring of your iodine levels, adjusting your intake as needed, and staying informed about the latest research will help you maintain the right balance for your body. With a proactive approach and a commitment to your well-being, thriving with iodine is within your reach, empowering you to lead a healthier, more energetic life.

Appendices and References

Appendix A: Food Sources of Iodine Chart

Seafood stands out as a powerhouse for iodine, with seaweed, such as kelp, nori, and wakame, leading the pack. These marine vegetables are not only versatile in culinary uses but also remarkably high in this essential nutrient. Fish, particularly cod and tuna, offer substantial amounts as well, making them excellent choices for those looking to boost their intake through diet.

Dairy products, including milk, cheese, and yogurt, are significant sources, thanks to the iodine supplements often given to cows and the disinfectant solutions used in dairy farming. The iodine content in dairy can vary depending on the farming practices and the animal's diet, but they generally provide a good contribution to the daily intake.

Eggs are another valuable contributor, with the iodine primarily located in the yolk. Chickens fed iodine-enriched feed produce eggs with higher levels of this nutrient, making them a convenient way to increase dietary intake.

Iodized salt, while a direct source of iodine, should be used judiciously. It can help prevent deficiency, especially in areas where other sources are scarce, but it's important to balance intake to avoid excessive sodium consumption.

Certain grains and cereals can also contribute to iodine intake, particularly those grown in iodine-rich soils. However, the amount can vary widely, so they should not be relied upon as the primary source.

Fruits and vegetables contain iodine, but the levels are dependent on the iodine content of the soil in which they are grown. Potatoes, cranberries, and strawberries are among those with higher levels, making them beneficial additions to a balanced diet.

It's crucial to note that while these food sources can help maintain adequate iodine levels, individual needs may vary, especially for those with specific health conditions or dietary restrictions. Consulting with a healthcare professional to tailor dietary choices to personal health requirements is always advisable.

Appendix B: Iodine Supplement Comparison Table

When evaluating iodine supplements, it's crucial to compare various aspects to determine the most suitable option for your health needs. Below is a detailed comparison table of different iodine supplements available on the market.

1. **Lugol's Solution**
   - **Type**: Liquid
   - **Iodine Content**: Approximately 6.3 mg per drop (2% solution)
   - **Additional Ingredients**: Potassium iodide
   - **Best For**: General use, adjustable dosing

2. **Nascent Iodine**
   - **Type**: Liquid
   - **Iodine Content**: About 400 mcg per drop
   - **Additional Ingredients**: Alcohol or vegetable glycerine as a base
   - **Best For**: Energy boost, easier absorption

3. **Potassium Iodide Tablets**
   - **Type**: Tablet
   - **Iodine Content**: Varies, commonly 130 mg per tablet
   - **Additional Ingredients**: Dicalcium phosphate, microcrystalline cellulose (binding agents)
   - **Best For**: Thyroid protection in radiation exposure

4. **Kelp Supplements**
   - **Type**: Capsule/Tablet
   - **Iodine Content**: Varies widely, often around 150-600 mcg per capsule
   - **Additional Ingredients**: May include fillers or other nutrients
   - **Best For**: Natural source, additional trace minerals

5. **Iodoral**
  - **Type**: Tablet
  - **Iodine Content**: 12.5 mg per tablet (combination of iodine and potassium iodide)
  - **Additional Ingredients**: Microsolle, a silica-based excipient
  - **Best For**: High-dose requirements, thyroid support

This comparison aims to provide a clear understanding of the options available, focusing on the form, iodine content, and unique benefits of each supplement. When choosing a supplement, consider your specific health goals, potential sensitivities to additional ingredients, and the advice of a healthcare professional.

Glossary: Iodine Terms and Concepts Explained

Autoimmune Thyroid Disorders: Conditions where the immune system mistakenly attacks the thyroid gland, leading to hypothyroidism (Hashimoto's thyroiditis) or hyperthyroidism (Graves' disease).

Bromide: A compound often found in commercial baked goods, soft drinks, and flame retardants, which can interfere with iodine absorption and thyroid function.

Detoxification (Detox): The process of removing toxic substances from the body. Iodine plays a role in detoxifying heavy metals and halides like fluoride and bromide.

Goiter: An enlargement of the thyroid gland, often due to iodine deficiency, which can lead to visible swelling in the neck.

Halides: A group of elements that includes fluoride, chloride, bromide, and iodide. Iodine is a beneficial halide, while the others can be disruptive to thyroid function when in excess.

Hyperthyroidism: A condition characterized by an overactive thyroid gland, leading to excessive production of thyroid hormones and symptoms like weight loss, anxiety, and rapid heartbeat.

Hypothyroidism: A condition where the thyroid gland is underactive, producing insufficient thyroid hormones, resulting in symptoms like fatigue, weight gain, and depression.

Iodine: A trace element essential for the production of thyroid hormones, which regulate metabolism, growth, and development.

Iodized Salt: Table salt that has been fortified with iodine to prevent deficiency. While helpful, it may not meet the body's entire iodine needs, especially in those with higher requirements or exposure to competing halides.

Lugol's Solution: A form of iodine solution that contains elemental iodine and potassium iodide, used as a supplement to support thyroid health and detoxification.

Nascent Iodine: A supplemental form of iodine, believed to be more bioavailable and gentle on the digestive system than other forms.

Selenium: A mineral that works synergistically with iodine to support thyroid function and protect against oxidative damage within the thyroid gland.

Thyroid Gland: A butterfly-shaped gland located in the neck, responsible for producing thyroid hormones that regulate metabolism, energy, and overall body function.

Made in United States
Troutdale, OR
03/13/2025

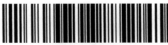

29737394R00069